Fundamentals of Oral and Maxillofacial Radiology

Fundamentals of Oral and Maxillofacial Radiology

J. Sean Hubar, DMD, MS
LSU School of Dentistry
New Orleans, LA, USA

With contributions by Paul Caballero

WILEY Blackwell

The right of J. Sean Hubar to be identified as the author of *Fundamentals of Oral and Maxillofacial Radiology* has been asserted in accordance with law.

Registered Offices
John Wiley & Sons, Inc., 111 River Street, Hoboken, NJ 07030, USA
John Wiley & Sons Ltd, The Atrium, Southern Gate, Chichester, West Sussex, PO19 8SQ, UK

Editorial Office
111 River Street, Hoboken, NJ 07030, USA

For details of our global editorial offices, customer services, and more information about Wiley products visit us at www.wiley.com.

Wiley also publishes its books in a variety of electronic formats and by print-on-demand. Some content that appears in standard print versions of this book may not be available in other formats.

Library of Congress Cataloging-in-Publication Data

Names: Hubar, J. Sean (Jack Sean), 1954– author.
Title: Fundamentals of oral and maxillofacial radiology / J. Sean Hubar.
Description: Hoboken, NJ : Wiley, 2017. | Includes bibliographical references and index.
Identifiers: LCCN 2017007878 (print) | LCCN 2017009355 (ebook) | ISBN 9781119122210 (paperback) |
    ISBN 9781119122234 (pdf) | ISBN 9781119122227 (epub)
Subjects: | MESH: Radiography, Dental
Classification: LCC RK309 (print) | LCC RK309 (ebook) | NLM WN 230 | DDC 617.6/07572–dc23
LC record available at https://lccn.loc.gov/2017007878

Cover images: left – courtesy of Adam Chen, XDR Radiology; middle and right – courtesy of J. Sean Hubar

Set in 9.5/12pt Palatino by SPi Global, Pondicherry, India
Printed and bound in Singapore by Markono Print Media Pte Ltd

10 9 8 7 6 5 4 3 2 1

Contents

☢ This symbol is used throughout this textbook to inform the reader that a definition of the adjacent italicized word (e.g. *barrier*) is defined in the Glossary of Terms section located toward the end of the book. It is actually the universal symbol for radiation that must be posted in public areas when ionizing radiation is in the immediate vicinity.

Acknowledgments

First, I would like to express my gratitude and appreciation to all those who have offered their assistance to me during the entire process of writing this book. In particular, I want to mention Holly for her love, total confidence and words of encouragement during the entire writing process. I would be remiss if I did not mention the three IT personnel at LSU School of Dentistry; Paul Caballero who contributed his talents to editing the text and digital images, Derrick Salvant for his technical contributions and Nick Funk for his technical skills and endless prodding that resulted in AFRB.

In addition, I want to thank my mentor, Dr. Kavas Thunthy, for his positive encouragement and Ms. Dale Hernandez for allowing me additional free time to pursue this project. I also am much obliged to the people at Wiley Publishers for allowing me to pursue this project and for their assistance.

Finally this book is dedicated to Jeffrey and to all those in the dental profession whom I hope benefit from reading this book.

J. Sean Hubar, DMD, MS

About the Companion Website

This book is accompanied by a companion website:

www.wiley.com/go/hubar/radiology

The website includes:
- PowerPoint files of all images from the book for downloading
- Spot the difference x-ray puzzles from Section T

Part One   Fundamentals

A Introduction

The objective of this textbook is to offer the reader a concise summary of the fundamentals and principles of dental radiology. In addition, brief synopses are included of the more common osseous pathologic lesions and dental anomalies. This book is intended to be a handy resource for the student, the dental auxiliary and the practicing clinician.

What is dental radiology?

Dental radiology is both an *art* and a *science*. An *art* is a skill acquired by experience, study or observation and a *science* is a technique that is tested through scientific method. Scientific principles of physics, chemistry, mathematics and biology are integral to dental radiology. Capturing and viewing a digital dental image requires sophisticated technology, while the operator's proper physical positioning of the intraoral receptor requires a skill that is based upon scientific principles. The art of dental radiology involves the interpretation of black and white images that often resemble ink blots. Deriving a differential diagnosis involves the application of the clinician's knowledge, cognitive skills and accumulated experience. The term "radiograph" originally applied to an x-ray

image made visible on a processed piece of x-ray film. A photograph is similar to a radiograph except it is taken with a light-sensitive camera and printed on photographic paper. Today the term "radiograph" is used to describe an image whether it was acquired with x-ray film or with a digital receptor. It is more accurate to use the term "x-ray image" when viewing it on a monitor and "digital radiograph" when a hardcopy is viewed. In the future, "radiograph" should be updated to a more appropriate term.

What are x rays?

X rays are a form of energy belonging to the electromagnetic (EM) spectrum. Some of the members of the EM family include radio waves, microwave radiation, infrared radiation, visible light, ultraviolet radiation, *x-ray radiation* and gamma radiation. These examples are differentiated by their wavelength and frequency. A *wavelength* is defined as the distance between two identical points on consecutive waves (e.g. distance from one crest to the next crest) (Fig. A1). Longer wavelengths have lower frequencies and are considered to be less damaging to living tissues. Conversely, shorter wavelengths

Fundamentals of Oral and Maxillofacial Radiology, First Edition. J. Sean Hubar.
© 2017 John Wiley & Sons, Inc. Published 2017 by John Wiley & Sons, Inc.
Companion website: www.wiley.com/go/hubar/radiology

have higher frequencies and are considered to be more damaging to living tissues. One end of the EM spectrum includes the long

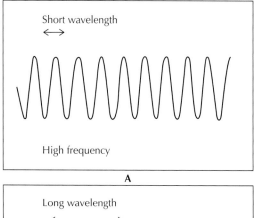

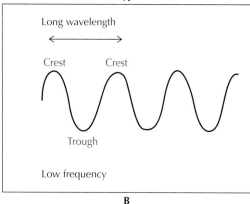

Fig. A1 Diagrams showing wave pattern of electromagnetic radiation. A. High frequency equals short wavelength. B. Low frequency equals long wavelength.

wavelengths used for radio signal communications while at the short wavelength end of the spectrum is gamma radiation. The EM spectrum covers wavelengths, ranging from *nanometers* to kilometers in length (Fig. A2). Dental x rays are 0.1 to 0.001 nanometers (nm) in length. For comparison purposes, dental x rays may be the size of a single atom while some radio waves are equivalent to the height of a tall building. As with all types of EM radiation, x rays are pure energy. They do not have any mass and because they have very short wavelengths, x rays can easily penetrate and potentially damage living tissues. All forms of EM radiation must not be confused with *particulate radiation*, such as *alpha* and *beta radiation*. Particulate radiation is not discussed in this textbook.

The EM spectrum is divided into the *non-ionizing* forms and the *ionizing* forms of radiation. The boundary between non-ionizing and ionizing radiation is not sharply delineated. Ionizing radiation is considered to begin with the shorter wavelength ultraviolet rays and the increasingly shorter wavelengths which include x rays and gamma rays. The longer wavelengths of ultraviolet rays and beyond which include microwaves, radio waves, etc. are all considered to be non-ionizing forms of radiation. The difference is that ionizing radiation is powerful enough to knock an *electron* out of its atomic orbit, while non-ionizing radiation is

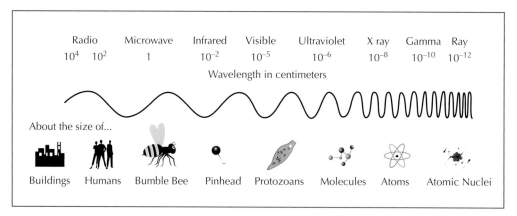

Fig. A2 Electromagnetic (EM) spectrum.

not powerful enough to remove an electron. The removal of an electron from an atom is referred to as "ionization." Exposure to ionizing radiation is recognized as being more hazardous to living tissue than non-ionizing radiation.

Note: "X ray" is actually a noun composed of two separate words and it should only be hyphenated when it is used as an adjective, e.g. *x-ray tube.* **In addition, each individual unit of electromagnetic radiation is referred to as a** *photon* ☢. **Consequently, the correct term for x ray is** *x-ray photon.* **In published literature, x-ray photons are often incorrectly referred to as "x-rays."**

In lay terms, x-ray images reveal the different parts of our bodies or other matter in varying shades of black and white. Why? This is because skin, bone, teeth, fat and air absorb different quantities of radiation. Within the human body, the calcium in bones and teeth absorbs the most x rays. Tooth enamel is the most mineralized substance in the human body (over 90% mineralized). Consequently, mineralized structures such as teeth and bones appear as varying shades of white (i.e. *radiopaque* ☢) on dental images. Fat and other soft tissues absorb less radiation, and consequently they will look darker (i.e. *radiolucent* ☢) in comparison to bone. Air absorbs the least amount of x rays, so airways and sinuses typically look black in comparison to mineralized substances. The denser or thicker the material, the more x-ray photons are absorbed by it. This results in a more radiopaque appearance on an x-ray image. The thinner or less dense an object is, the fewer the number of x-ray photons absorbed or blocked by it. Thus more x-ray photons are able to penetrate through the object to expose the image recording receptor. This results in a more radiolucent appearance.

What's the big deal about x-ray images?

Just as the early pioneers in radiology were astonished to see the previously unknown in their first x-ray images, modern day clinicians may be astonished to see osseous and dental pathology, anatomic variations, effects of trauma, etc. on their x-ray images. Consequently, the benefits of x-ray images are immense. The combination of both clinical and x-ray images provides vital information to the dentist for preparing comprehensive dental treatment plans. The end result is a continual improvement in oral healthcare today.

B History

Discovery of x rays

On November 8, 1895, *Wilhelm Konrad Röntgen* (alternately spelled Wilhelm Conrad Roentgen), a professor of physics and the director of the Physical Institute of the Julius Maximilian University at Würzburg in Germany, while working in his laboratory discovered what we commonly call "x rays" (Fig. B1). On that day in his darkened laboratory, he noticed light emanating on a table located across the room, far from the experiment that he was conducting. Professor Röntgen was researching the effects of electrical discharge using a *Crookes–Hittorf tube* ☢. The glowing object was a fluorescent screen used in another experiment. This perplexed him because electrons emanating from his electric discharge tube were known to only travel short distances in air. His fluorescing screen was too far away for these electrons to produce the fluorescence. In addition, his lab was completely darkened and the Crookes–Hittorf tube was completely covered with black cardboard to prevent light leakage. Light leakage otherwise could have caused the screen to fluoresce. It was obvious to Professor Röntgen that he was dealing with an unknown invisible phenomenon. Professor Röntgen called this new phenomenon "x rays." "X" because that is

the universal symbol for the unknown and "ray" because it traveled in a straight line. He was a modest gentleman and did not wish to call these new rays "Röntgen rays" after himself which is standard protocol for new discoveries. Following his discovery of x rays, he was determined to learn what were the properties and characteristics of these mysterious invisible rays. He secretly tested this phenomenon for weeks and did not divulge any information about his new discovery to anyone. At first he experimented by placing objects in the path of the x rays between the tube and the fluorescent screen. Ultimately, he decided to place his own hand in front of the x-ray beam and he was amazed at what he saw on the fluorescent screen. He observed shadows of his skin and underlying bones. For the first recorded image, he asked his wife, Bertha, to place her hand on a photographic plate while he operated the experimental apparatus. Professor Röntgen was able to produce an x-ray image of her bones and soft tissue. This x-ray image, which includes the wedding ring on her finger, is recognized as the first *x-ray image* of the human body (Fig. B2).

On December 28, 1895, Professor Röntgen delivered his first of three manuscripts on x rays to the president of the Physical Medical

Fundamentals of Oral and Maxillofacial Radiology, First Edition. J. Sean Hubar.
© 2017 John Wiley & Sons, Inc. Published 2017 by John Wiley & Sons, Inc.
Companion website: www.wiley.com/go/hubar/radiology

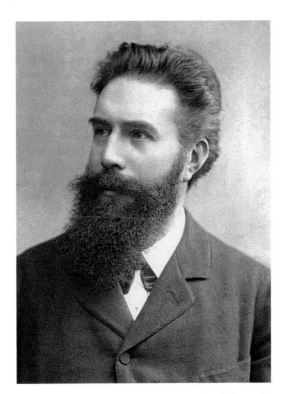

Fig. B1 Wilhelm Konrad Röntgen: credited with being the first person to discover x rays.

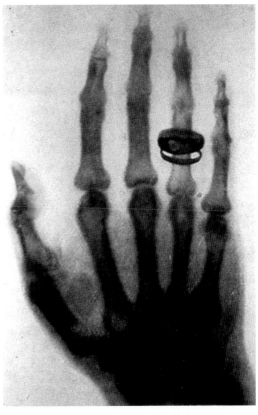

Fig. B2 First x-ray image of the human body: Bertha Röntgen's hand.

Society of Würzburg. The first manuscript was entitled "On a New Kind of Rays, A Preliminary Communication." The unedited manuscript went to press immediately and was published in the *Annals of the Society*. Immediately afterwards, announcements were published in newspapers and in scientific journals around the world. In the United States, the announcement of Professor Röntgen's discovery was on January 7, 1896 in the *New York Herald* newspaper. The English translations of the original paper were printed in *Nature,* a London publication, on January 23, 1896 and in *Science,* a New York publication, on February 14, 1896. Professor Röntgen did not seek nor enjoy public acclaim and as a result he would make only a single presentation on the topic of x rays. This presentation was given to the Physical Medical Society of Würzburg on January 23, 1896.

The prevalence of *Ruhmkorff coils* ☢ and Crookes–Hittorf tubes in nearly every physics laboratory at the time permitted x-ray research to be conducted globally without much delay. These two ingredients were the primary components necessary for producing x rays. Consequently, prior to Professor Röntgen's discovery anyone who was studying high voltage electricity was unknowingly generating x rays. But no one prior to Professor Röntgen recognized this phenomenon, nor understood the value of it even if they did suspect something unusual. Sir William Crookes, whose collaboration produced the Crookes–Hittorf tubes, had outright complained to the manufacturer that unopened boxes of photographic plates were arriving at his lab already exposed. Sir Crookes surmised the problem was simply due to the manufacturer's poor quality control. It was not until after Professor Röntgen's discovery was announced that Sir Crookes and other scientists finally understood that x rays were the cause of some of their photographic plate problems.

Professor Röntgen was awarded the first Nobel Prize for Physics in 1901 for his discovery of x rays even though some tried to discredit his claim to the discovery. Sadly, Professor Röntgen became reclusive and very bitter in his later years as a result of this controversy concerning the discovery of x rays. He even stipulated in his will that all of his correspondences written regarding the discovery of x rays be destroyed at his death. He died on February 10, 1923. Unbeknownst to Professor Röntgen, his recognition of x rays is considered by many today to be the greatest scientific discovery of all time. X rays have truly revolutionized modern healthcare practices.

Who took the world's first "dental" radiograph?

Poor records make it difficult to say conclusively who took the first dental radiograph. However, Professor Walter König in Frankfurt, Germany, Dr. Otto Walkoff, a dentist in Brunschweig, Germany and Dr. Frank Harrison, a dentist in Sheffield, England have all been reported to have taken dental radiographs within a month of Röntgen 's reported discovery. Dr. Walkoff on January 14, 1896 used a glass photographic plate. The glass plate was wrapped in black paper to block out light and it was covered with rubber dam to keep out saliva. He inserted this glass plate into his own mouth and subjected himself to a 25 min exposure to radiation (Fig. B3). If not the first dental radiograph, it certainly was one of the earliest dental radiographs. Most people claim that Dr. C. Edmund Kells, Jr. took the *first dental radiograph of a living person in the United States*. It should be emphasized that this was on a *living person* because it had been reported earlier in a *Dental*

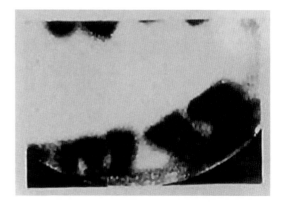

Fig. B3 First *dental* radiograph (unconfirmed). In January 1896, Dr. Otto Walkoff, a German dentist, covered a small glass photographic plate and wrapped it in a rubber sheath. He then positioned it in his mouth and subsequently exposed himself to 25 min of radiation.

Cosmos publication that Dr. Wm. J. Morton, a physician, presented his research work before the New York Odontological Society and it included four dental x-ray radiographs. But his dental radiographs were taken on dried laboratory skulls and not on a living person. According to Dr. Kells, "Just when I took my first dental radiograph, I cannot say, because I have no record of it, but in the transactions of the Southern Dental Association, there is reported my x-ray clinic given in Asheville in July 1896, and I remember full well that I had had the apparatus several months before giving this clinic and had developed a method of taking dental radiographs. Thus I must have begun work in April or May 1896." Regardless of who was first to expose a dental radiograph, the value of dental radiography was recognized almost immediately after Professor Röntgen's discovery of x rays.

Dr. C. E. Kells, Jr., a New Orleans dentist and the early days of dental radiography

Shortly after the announcement of Professor Röntgen's discovery, Professor Brown Ayres of Tulane University in New Orleans gave a public demonstration of x rays using a crude apparatus set-up. Since the general public marveled at the thought of being able to stand next to a piece of equipment and shortly thereafter see a photograph of the inside of the body, he devoted a portion of his demonstration to expose a volunteer's hand. Although it required a lengthy 20 min exposure, the crowd was patient, including one curious soul, Dr. C. Edmund Kells, Jr. (Fig. B4). It immediately occurred to him that x rays would be an invaluable tool for observing inside the jaws and teeth. Dr. Kells met Professor Ayres and they discussed the idea of taking pictures of teeth. Professor Ayres became instrumental in assisting Kells to acquire the necessary equipment for building an x-ray laboratory to conduct his own research.

It was a crude and difficult procedure for taking x rays in the early days. For example, one of the original problems encountered was the variability in output of the x-ray tube. The few molecules of air that were inside the tube were vital for producing x rays. To do so, some

of these air molecules would have to be bombarded into the walls of the tube, which would convert their energy into x rays. The air molecules received that energy when a very high voltage was supplied to the tube. In doing this, however, these molecules of air would gradually adhere to the inner walls of the tube and without any free air molecules present floating inside the tube, x rays could not be produced. To reverse this situation, the x-ray tube would have to be heated by means of an alcohol lamp. The heat would drive the air molecules off the walls, allowing x rays to be produced once again. The constantly changing conditions within the tube meant that the apparatus had to be reset for each and every patient. Otherwise, there was no way of determining how long a photographic plate would need to be exposed to get a good image.

To complicate matters further, meters were not available in the early days to measure exactly how much radiation was being produced by the x-ray apparatus. The accepted method of choice was for a clinician, such as Dr. Kells, to pick up a fluoroscope and place one hand in front of it. The radiation output would be adjusted until the bones of the hand were visible in the fluoroscope. An equally hazardous technique would be for the operator to place a hand in front of the beam and adjust the radiation output until the skin began to turn red. This is referred to as the *erythema dose* ☢. The patient would then be positioned in front of the x-ray beam and the exposure taken. The absence of any immediate accompanying sensation by the patient frequently led to radiation overexposure. Furthermore, the clinician was in close proximity to the patient during the entire exposure and was completely unshielded.

Dr. Kells immediately could foresee several problems with incorporating x rays into a dental practice. His primary concern was the exposure time. If it took 20 min for a hand to be exposed, it theoretically might require hours to expose a tooth because a tooth is a much denser object. How could a patient hold a

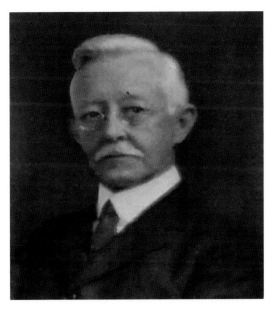

Fig. B4 Dr. C. Edmund Kells, Jr.: New Orleans dentist, inventor and author.

dental x-ray film motionless for that length of time? Dr. Kells' early trials showed that it would require up to 15 min to expose a molar tooth, which was much better than he anticipated, but it still was a monumental problem to overcome. If dental x rays were to be routinely taken by the dental practitioner, technical improvements to reduce time exposures were crucial. Within three years of Professor Röntgen's discovery rapid improvements in the design of the x-ray tube dramatically reduced that 15 min exposure down to 1–2 min. Then there was a major alteration in the tube design on May 12, 1913. This was the patent application date for the *Coolidge tube* and this ushered in the "golden age of radiology." W. O. Coolidge, the director of research at the General Electric Company, found that using a coil of tungsten in a low vacuum tube could generate significantly more x rays than the old gas style tubes could ever produce. As a result, in the 1920s x-ray exposures were dramatically reduced to 4–10 s in duration.

There were also electrical dangers. An uninsulated and unprotected wire carried a high voltage current to the discharge tube which led to injuries to both patients and clinicians. In 1917, Henry Fuller Waite, Jr. patented the design for an x-ray unit that eliminated the exposed high voltage wire. General Electric introduced the Victor CDX shockproof dental x-ray unit about a year later.

All x-ray demonstrations on human patients initially used large glass plates for recording the images. It was not until 1919 that the first machine-wrapped dental x-ray film packet became commercially available. It was called *regular film* and was manufactured by the Eastman Kodak Company. Now that x-ray film was small enough to place inside a patient's mouth, how were patients supposed to hold it in place and keep it steady? To overcome both these problems, Dr. Kells produced his own rubber film holder with a pocket in it for holding the film. The side of the film holder was made of an aluminum plate and the wrapped film was placed in the pocket. With the patient's mouth closed, the film holder was held in place by the opposing teeth. He selected one of his dental assistants to be his subject. This person is regarded as being the first living person in the United States to have experienced a dental x-ray exposure. She sat in a dental chair with the film holder in place with her face placed up against the side of a thin board. In this manner, she was able to hold perfectly still for the required time. Unbeknownst to Dr. Kells at the time, using the thin board acted as an x-ray filter that helped to prevent his assistant from receiving a radiation burn to her face from the prolonged exposure. Filters eventually would become a standard feature in all modern x-ray units.

Just as there were extravagant claims made for using x rays for the eradication of facial blemishes such as birth-marks and moles, removal of unwanted hair and curing cancer, early advocates met with considerable opposition to the diagnostic use of x rays and it often came from within the profession. Not only did they oppose the use of x rays, they openly condemned it. Dr. John S. Marshall in June of 1897 told the members of the Section on Stomatology of the American Medical Association that he had intended to use the rays in his practice, but had been deterred by the danger. Tragically, many early pioneers eventually developed fatal cancers from exposure to tremendous amounts of accumulated radiation received in monitoring and operating the x-ray apparatus. Dr. Kells himself developed cancer that was attributed to radiation exposure. Even so, he stated in the last article he wrote "Do I murmur at the rough deal the fates have dealt me? No, I can't do that. When I think of the thousands of suffering patients who are benefited every day by the use of x rays, I cannot complain. That a few suffer for the benefits of the millions is a law of nature." Sadly, after years of suffering and failed medical treatments, he committed suicide in his dental office in 1928.

C Generation of X Rays

X rays occur in nature (e.g. solar x rays) but dental x rays are strictly a man-made entity. Dental x-ray equipment is manufactured by multiple companies, each offering varying styles, sizes, features and prices for their own particular units. The physical dental x-ray unit primarily consists of two components. There is a control panel with a circuit board to control the *kilovoltage (kV)* ☢, *milliamperage (mA)* ☢ and time. In addition, there is a tubehead that physically houses the x-ray tube, filter, collimator and *transformers* ☢ (Fig. C1). The tubehead and control panel may be physically separate (e.g. wall-mounted x-ray unit) or they may be combined (e.g. hand-held x-ray unit). Individual mA and kV controls are features that vary from one unit to another. Higher quality x-ray units tend to have independent controls to modify the kV, mA and exposure time while basic intraoral units may have fixed or a very limited number of mA and kV settings that an operator may alter. All intraoral x-ray units allow the operator to modify the exposure time. Extraoral x-ray units (eg. panoramic) generate x rays in a similar way to intraoral x-ray units but are physically very different.

The heart of an x-ray unit is the x-ray tube (Fig. C2). An x-ray tube primarily consists of a *cathode* ☢ and an *anode* ☢. The operator's simple act of powering on a dental x-ray unit (i.e. on–off switch) sends a low voltage current to the cathode which results in the production of a cloud of electrons at the cathode. The x-ray unit is in a stand-by mode at this time.

When it is time to expose the intraoral x-ray image, the operator must press an exposure button. Pressing the exposure button will convert standard wall outlet electricity to a high voltage current via a step-up transformer and send it directly to the x-ray tube. A *step-up* transformer is the actual device that boosts the voltage high enough for x-ray production. The effect of this high voltage is that it accelerates the electrons from the cathode across the tube to the anode. The anode is composed of a copper stem and a smaller target area composed of tungsten. The tungsten target area is referred to as a focal spot. The purpose of the copper stem is to assist dissipating the heat generated when electrons strike the focal spot, thereby extending the useful life of the x-ray tube. Once these energized electrons accelerate across the tube and strike the focal spot, only about 1% of the resulting *kinetic energy* ☢ is converted into x rays, while the remaining 99% of the energy is converted into heat. Oil fills the tubehead to act as an electrical insulator and helps to dissipate the heat generated from x-ray production.

Fundamentals of Oral and Maxillofacial Radiology, First Edition. J. Sean Hubar.
© 2017 John Wiley & Sons, Inc. Published 2017 by John Wiley & Sons, Inc.
Companion website: www.wiley.com/go/hubar/radiology

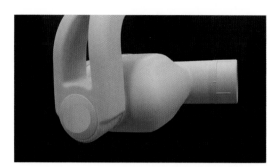

Fig. C1 Dental x-ray tubehead.

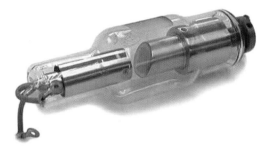

Fig. C2 X-ray tube.

A step-up transformer may generate voltages upwards of 120 kV. Modern day intraoral x-ray units typically operate in the 60–70 kV range; extraoral dental x-ray units generally require voltages up to 120 kV. There is also a *step-down*

transformer located within the confines of the tubehead. The step-down transformer reduces the voltage from a standard household electrical outlet to approximately 8–10 V. This low voltage is then sent to the filament of the cathode, which produces an *electron cloud* ☢ that will be used to produce our dental x-rays. Reducing the voltage to the cathode filament also extends the useful life of the x-ray unit. The cathode filament and anode focal spot typically are both made of tungsten. Obviously a 1% production rate for an x-ray unit is a very inefficient use of electricity, but it generates adequate amounts of x radiation for our dental needs. With normal office usage, dental x-ray units will last many years.

Note: At the end of the working day, both intraoral and extraoral x-ray units should be powered off. Keeping an x-ray unit powered on indefinitely results in a continuous flow of current to the x-ray tube, thereby shortening the useful life of that tube. Unlike intraoral and panoramic x-ray units, when a cone beam computed tomographic unit is powered down overnight it will typically need upwards of 30 min for the flat panel receptor to properly warm-up again prior to taking the first patient exposure.

D Exposure Controls

Figure D1 shows an x-ray control panel displaying variable exposure parameters.

Voltage (V)

Voltage controls the penetrability of the x-ray beam and the degree of *contrast* ☢ in the image. One kilovolt (kV) is equivalent to 1000 V. When exposing intraoral images, selecting a higher kilovoltage increases the number of shades of gray between black and white in the image. This is referred to as a *lower contrast* image. This is particularly useful for diagnosing periodontal issues where varying bone level heights are a concern. Higher kilovoltage also is useful for imaging maxillary posterior teeth where the patient's alveolar ridge and soft tissue thickness are typically greater. Additionally, increasing the penetrability of the x-ray beam through superimposing osseous structures, such as the zygoma, will improve the diagnostic quality of the image. Meanwhile a lower kilovoltage exposure setting reduces the number of shades of gray in the intraoral image. This is referred to as a *higher contrast* image. This is particularly useful for detecting caries. This benefits the clinician who wishes to only differentiate between healthy tooth structure and decayed tooth structure. On both intraoral and extraoral dental images, tooth decay will appear *radiolucent*.

Amperage (A)

Amperage primarily controls the quantity of x rays generated. Dental units use milliamperes (mA). One milliampere is one-thousandth of an *ampere* ☢. Amperage controls the number of electrons in the cloud that will ultimately travel across the x-ray tube, hit the anode and produce x-ray photons. A basic dental x-ray unit typically has a single milliamperage setting, while a higher quality x-ray unit will have multiple millamperage settings. Intraoral x-ray units generally produce 4–15 mA. Selecting a higher milliamperage will increase the number of x rays generated and result in an overall denser (i.e. darker) x-ray image. If an initial x-ray image appears too dark, reducing the milliamperage for a follow-up exposure will lighten the overall density of the new image.

Fundamentals of Oral and Maxillofacial Radiology, First Edition. J. Sean Hubar.
© 2017 John Wiley & Sons, Inc. Published 2017 by John Wiley & Sons, Inc.
Companion website: www.wiley.com/go/hubar/radiology

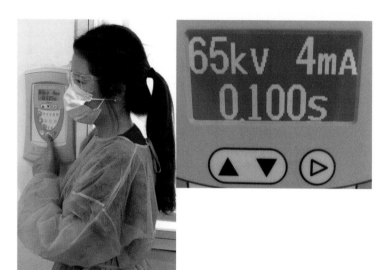

Fig. D1 X-ray control panel displaying variable kilovoltage (kV), milli-amperage (mA) and time settings.

Exposure timer

All intraoral dental x-ray units must include an exposure timer to control the duration of radiation production. Modern digital timers are capable of expressing time in thousandths of a second. Some manufacturers' timers use "number of impulses" not "fractions of a second" as exposure increments. However, impulses can easily be converted into seconds. Impulses are associated with the electrical frequency (i.e. number of hertz). To convert impulses into seconds, simply divide the number of impulses by the number of *hertz (Hz)* ☢. In North America, standard household electric current is 60 Hz (cycles per second), while in Europe it is 50 Hz. Selecting a 30 impulse time would translate into an exposure of 0.5 s (30 impulses divided by 60) in the United States. The function of altering the exposure time permits adapting to different patient types (e.g. physical size, gagging reflex, etc.) to achieve optimal image quality. Increasing the exposure time will result in the generation of more x rays and consequently produce an overall denser (i.e. darker) x-ray image. Conversely, a shorter time of exposure will result in a less dense (i.e. lighter) x-ray image. In general, image contrast is not affected by exposure time.

E

Radiation Dosimetry

The terminology used to differentiate radiation doses includes: (i) absorbed dose; (ii) equivalent dose; and (iii) effective dose. The **international system of units** (abbreviated **SI** from the French derivation *Le Système Internationale d'Unités*) is the modern form of the metric system and is the world's most widely used system of radiation measurement, used in both everyday commerce and science (see Appendix 6).

Exposure

Exposure refers to the radiation output of an x-ray machine. It is a measure of the ionization in air produced by x rays or gamma rays. *Roentgen (R)* ☢ is the traditional unit of measure. The SI term that is the equivalent of a roentgen is *coulombs per kilogram*. One roentgen is equivalent to 2.58×10^{-4} C/kg.

Absorbed dose

Radiation absorbed dose (rad) quantifies the energy from x radiation that is absorbed by a given mass of tissue. This is the numeric difference between how much x radiation enters and how much x radiation exits a mass of tissue. The SI unit for absorbed dose is called a *gray* (Gy). The conversion rate is 1 Gy equals 100 rad.

Equivalent dose

Clinical dentistry is typically limited to using one type of radiation, "x rays." However, the general public is continually exposed to a variety of types of radiation during a lifetime, whether it is medical or environmental in origin. *Equivalent dose* is a measure specifically used to compare the biologic effects of different types of radiation on living tissues. The biologic effects due to different types of radiation are significant. The SI unit for equivalent dose is *sievert (Sv)* ☢. The original unit for equivalent dose was referred to as a *rem*, which is an acronym for *radiation equivalent man (rem)* ☢. Similar to converting rad units to gray units, the conversion is 1 Sv equals 100 rem.

Note: In clinical dentistry, the terms *rads*, *rems*, *grays* and *sieverts* are often used interchangeably when discussing patient exposures. However, when a researcher wishes to conduct a scientific study, using the precise nomenclature is critical.

Fundamentals of Oral and Maxillofacial Radiology, First Edition. J. Sean Hubar.
© 2017 John Wiley & Sons, Inc. Published 2017 by John Wiley & Sons, Inc.
Companion website: www.wiley.com/go/hubar/radiology

Effective dose

Different cell types may react differently to an identical dose of x-radiation exposure (e.g. muscle cell versus erythrocyte cell). *Effective dose* ☢ takes into account the differences in cellular response from radiation. It is also useful for comparing risks from different imaging procedures (e.g. dental imaging versus medical imaging) because it factors into account the absorbed dose to all body organs, the relative harm from radiation and the sensitivities of each organ to radiation. As a result, effective dose is a good indicator of the possible long-term radiation risks to the individual.

F

Radiation Biology

Shortly after the discovery of x radiation, adverse effects of radiation exposure were being observed. The cellular effects would begin with erythema, followed by dermatitis, ulceration and ultimately the growth of tumors. All of which are associated with increasing amounts of radiation exposure. Pioneers in the dental field were ignorant of the hazards of radiation and some clinicians required amputations of fingers as a result of excessive radiation exposure from holding the image receptors in their patients' mouths.

The time lag between an individual's exposure to radiation and the observed effect of the radiation is called the *latent period*. The latent period may be a very brief period as in the time it takes for a sunburn to become visible. Sunburn is caused by an excessive skin exposure to ultraviolet radiation in a relatively short period of time. The reddening of the skin typically appears several hours after exposure to the sun. This is considered to be a short latent period. At the opposite end, we do not have a defined maximum length of time for an effect to be observed. A latent period may require decades or generations before an effect is ultimately observed. Why? Because x-radiation damage to an individual's *germ cells* ♠♠ (i.e. sperm and ova), will not be observed in the exposed individual. Rather, the radiation

effects will be observed in the affected individual's future offspring. Because of this, the offspring of the survivors of the 1945 Hiroshima and Nagasaki atomic bombings continue to be followed today for possible long-term genetic effects.

Currently, we do not know the long-term effects from low doses of radiation. One reason for why the effects of low-dose radiation exposure are still unknown is because individuals cannot be ethically studied in a controlled environment where a researcher can completely monitor and control a person's day to day lifestyle. Lifestyle factors include diet, vocation, home environment and chronic habits such as smoking, etc. All of these lifestyle choices can deleteriously affect an individual's long-term health and cloud the effects of radiation alone. Consequently, with uncertainty as to the effects of low-dose radiation, all precautions to reduce unnecessary exposure to both the patient and the operator should be followed (see Section G).

Biologic effects of radiation are classified as either a *direct* or an *indirect effect*. If an incoming x-ray photon modifies a biologic molecule, it is called a *direct effect* (e.g. break in a chromosomal chain). However, when the biologic effect is the result of a subsequent intermediary change to a molecule, the effect is termed an *indirect effect*.

Fundamentals of Oral and Maxillofacial Radiology, First Edition. J. Sean Hubar.
© 2017 John Wiley & Sons, Inc. Published 2017 by John Wiley & Sons, Inc.
Companion website: www.wiley.com/go/hubar/radiology

Water being the predominate molecule of a living human, it is frequently affected by ionizing radiation. An incoming x-ray photon may hydrolyze (i.e. split) a water molecule. This first action is a *direct effect* of radiation. However, following the hydrolysis of water, there may be a recombination of the byproducts, hydroperoxyl and hydrogen, which can produce a molecule of an organic hydrogen peroxide. This would be an *indirect effect* of radiation. This organic hydrogen peroxide molecule can lead to cell death or a future mutation of the cell. Overall, direct effects of radiation account for approximately 33% of all biologic damage, while the remaining 67% of biologic damage is the result of indirect effects. Tissue sensitivity to radiation varies depending upon the tissue type (see Effective dose in Section E).

What happens to the dental x-ray photons that are directed at a patient?

X rays can pass through unchanged

The relative vastness of space in the atom separating electrons and the infinitesimally small size of each x-ray photon permits a small percentage of x-ray photons to pass directly through the atom without any interaction, possibly up to 10% of the total dose. In practice, the patient is typically positioned between the x-ray tubehead and the operator. Since we know that 100% of the x-ray beam is not absorbed by the patient, it is imperative that the operator not stand directly in-line with the beam of x-radiation (see Section G).

X rays can undergo a coherent scatter

Coherent scatter (aka Thompson scatter) occurs rarely when a low energy incoming x-ray photon collides with an outer shell electron of an atom. The photon does not have enough energy to eject that electron from its orbit. The net result is: (i) no

net change to the atom; (ii) the incoming x-ray photon loses some of its energy upon impact with the electron; and (iii) the x-ray photon is redirected (i.e. scattered). This x-ray photon will continue interacting with other atoms until all of its energy is dissipated. These redirected x-ray photons are called *scattered x rays*. Even though the scatter dose is low, this author recommends that the operator should place a protective apron on every patient and that the operator should stand behind a protective barrier during an x-ray exposure. These are simple methods to reduce the effects of scatter radiation for both the patient and the operator. Further reducing radiation exposure to both the patient and the operator when feasible is still the best principle.

X rays can produce a photoelectric effect

Photoelectric effect accounts for upwards of 25% of x-ray interactions. The incoming x-ray photon collides and is absorbed entirely by an inner shell electron. This incoming photon imparts enough energy to the electron so that together they are ejected from its orbit. This ejected electron is now called a *photoelectron* (i.e. photon+electron=photoelectron). This photoelectron travels short distances before giving up all of its energy during additional collisions. Within the same atom, another electron from a higher orbit may drop into the void created by the photoelectron. In so doing, it generates an additional low energy x-ray photon, referred to as a *characteristic* or *secondary* x ray. Secondary x-ray photons do not benefit the patient or the clinician. They are generally absorbed by the patient's soft tissues but they also can produce image *fog* ☢. Secondary x rays pose no external threat to the operator.

X rays can produce a Compton scatter

Compton scatter accounts for the majority of interactions with dental x-ray photons. In this scenario, an incoming x-ray photon has sufficient energy to knock out an outer shell electron. The result is a redirection of the incoming x-ray photon after it collides with an electron and the formation of an *ion pair*. An ion pair consists of a negatively-charged ejected electron and the resultant positively-charged atom. The term *ionizing radiation* is applied to this phenomenon. X rays are classified as a form of ionizing radiation. Both the ejected electron and the weakened scattered x-ray photon can continue to interact with other atoms. This can result in additional ionizations and with each ensuing impact the x-ray photon will continue to be weakened while other atoms attempting to reach a state of maximum stability will seek out the recoil electron.

Determinants of biologic damage from x-radiation exposure

Exposure dose

Any amount of ionizing radiation will produce some biologic damage. Regardless of how minute the radiation exposure dose may be, there will always be some long-term residual damage to the radiated area. Minimal residual damage may not be visible initially. However, after repeated exposures to ionizing radiation, termed *chronic exposure*, a biologic effect will ultimately present itself. This classification of cellular response is referred to as a *deterministic effect* ☢. The total amount of radiation exposure required to elicit a cellular effect is called the *threshold dose* ☢. Below the threshold level of exposure, no effect will be observed. A simple example of a threshold radiation dose effect is sunburn. Acute biologic effects from increasing doses of ionizing begin with erythema, followed by dermatitis, ulceration, tanning and ultimately the loss of glandular function. Erythema occurs after exposure to approximately 250 cGy of radiation that is delivered in a relatively short span (e.g. two weeks). In comparison, a dental bitewing exposure is minimal

at approximately 0.08 µGy. A second type of biologic effect of ionizing radiation is called a *stochastic effect* ☢. In this classification, either the effect occurs or it does not occur – it is an all or nothing response. Cancer is an example of a stochastic effect. Individuals do not develop a mild case of cancer or a severe case of cancer. They are all cancers.

In dentistry, exposure dose is affected by variable factors that include the distance of the x-ray source from the face, kilovoltage, milliamperage and exposure time. All these factors combined will determine the total radiation dose to the patient.

Note: It is extremely important for all of us to remember that although the biologic effects resulting from high doses of radiation exposure are known, the long-term effects from low doses of ionizing radiation are still unknown. This is why we need to refrain from exposing individuals to any unnecessary imaging procedures whenever possible or, at the very least, utilize a projection that requires a minimum of radiation exposure. In addition, the operator should take all precautions to minimize their own exposure to radiation while performing imaging procedures.

Dose rate

The time interval between repeated exposures to ionizing radiation influences the extent of biologic damage. A rapid rate of recurring radiation exposure with minimal time between each exposure will result in more biologic damage than if an equal cumulative radiation dose (i.e. total dose) was administered over a longer time frame. Incremental doses of radiation are preferable because it permits the body time to repair some of the biologic damage before the next dose is administered. Multiple smaller doses of radiation administered over an extended time interval allows greater cellular repair. Conversely, a high dose of radiation administered in a single session diminishes a body's ability to recuperate and repair the non-cancerous cells. A skin tan is a threshold effect that occurs from gradual cumulative doses of ultraviolet radiation versus a sunburn effect that results from a single concentrated dose of ultraviolet radiation. But to be clear, the ultraviolet "tan" effect is still biologic damage to the individual's skin, but just not as severe as a sunburn effect. We also know that individuals with years of repeated ultraviolet skin damage have a greater incidence of basal cell or squamous cell carcinomas.

Area of exposure

The volume of tissue exposed to radiation plays a significant role in the overall well-being of the patient. Patients receiving localized oral cancer radiotherapy, possibly up to 70 Gy, may encounter severe biologic effects in the irradiated field that often will culminate in the loss of glandular function and *osteoradionecrosis* ☢☢. However, total exposure to a much lower dose of 3–5 Gy administered over the entire body would very likely result in death of the individual. Whole body radiation affects all of the body's biologic systems simultaneously and, as a result, the body's attempt to repair cellular damage is overwhelmed. Consequently, death of an individual will occur from far less whole body radiation exposure compared with administering a mega dose of radiation that is concentrated to a localized area.

Current guidelines from the National Council on Radiation Protection and Measurements (NCRP) stipulate that rectangular collimation shall be used for periapical and bitewing imaging and should be used for occlusal imaging when possible. Rectangular collimation shall also be used with hand-held devices whenever possible and x-ray equipment for cephalometric imaging shall provide for asymmetric collimation of the beam to the area of clinical interest. All of these NCRP guidelines

are made to reduce the area of radiation exposure to the patient.

Age

All living beings are susceptible to the effects of x radiation. However, younger and older individuals are most susceptible. High metabolic rates in younger individuals and the poor recuperative healing powers in older individuals result in greater risks from radiation exposure. This does not eliminate the intermediate age group from experiencing ill effects from ionizing radiation, it only means that this age group is less susceptible to the effects. Precautions to reduce exposure to ionizing radiation apply to all age groups. NCRP recommendations for pediatric patients include: (i) select x rays for individual needs; (ii) use the fastest image receptor possible; (iii) collimate the beam to the area of interest; (iv) always use a thyroid collar unless it interferes with imaging the needed anatomy; and (v) use cone beam computed tomography (CBCT) only when necessary.

Cell type

The *Law of Bergonie and Tribondeau* of 1906 states that the most radiation-sensitive cells types are undifferentiated, divide quickly and are highly active metabolically. Amongst the most sensitive cell types are erythrocytes and stem cells. Among the least sensitive cell types are neural and muscle cells. Two exceptions to the law are oocytes and lymphocytes. These two varieties are very specialized cell types and they are very sensitive to radiation. It is not clear as to why these two cell types are particularly sensitive to radiation.

Pioneers in dental radiology were ignorant of the dangers of x radiation and many suffered the consequences of excessive exposure. Dental exposure doses today are considered to be very low in comparison. However, as stated earlier, any amount of exposure to ionizing radiation produces some cellular damage. Although a carcinoma is statistically unlikely to result from dental x rays, theoretically it could result from the minute amount of radiation exposure used to produce a single dental image. Consequently, exposing patients to any amount of x radiation should be limited and imaging should only be ordered when it is vital for diagnosing the patient's oral health.

G

Radiation Protection

Very soon after x rays were discovered, it became apparent that x rays were harmful. As early as 1897, there were cases of skin damage. In 1901, a pioneer in dentistry, *William H. Rollins, DDS, MD*, observed that x rays could cause tissue burns and attempted to warn dentists and physicians of the dangers of x rays. Little heed was taken of Dr. Rollins warnings but, shortly after, the dental profession began to take measures to reduce the damaging effects of radiation. However, many pioneers in dentistry, whether through ignorance or neglect, suffered the loss of one or more fingers because they repeatedly held the x-ray film used to record the dental image in the patient's mouth. X-ray film was the standard for recording dental images at the time.

Utilization of radiation in a dental office requires regulations to protect the patient, the operator and any employees or bystanders located within the working environment. *ALARA* is an acronym for "**a**s **l**ow **a**s **r**easonably **a**chievable." If the exposure dose to a patient can be easily reduced, then it should be. The ALARA principle is recognized by the American Dental Association (ADA) and is expected to be followed by dental practitioners. Because of concerns today about the overutilization of ionizing radiation procedures in medicine, ALARA is morphing into ALADA. *ALADA* ☢ is an acronym for "**a**s **l**ow **a**s **d**iagnostically **a**cceptable." Reducing the exposure dose to a patient to a minimum, yet still being able to diagnose the images, is beginning to be practiced in the medical community and should be adopted in dentistry as well.

Quality assurance (QA) refers to optimized dental images produced with minimum radiation exposure. Minimum exposure to radiation applies not only to the patient, but also the dental operator and any bystanders in proximity to the dental x-ray equipment. The ADA and NCRP set guidelines that every dental healthcare setting adopts regarding maintaining x-ray equipment, image receptors, protective aprons, etc.

1. RADIATION PROTECTION: PATIENT

Protecting the patient entails both reducing the exposure dose from the primary x-ray beam that is directed at the patient's head and the subsequent scatter radiation that may affect other regions of the body.

Fundamentals of Oral and Maxillofacial Radiology, First Edition. J. Sean Hubar.
© 2017 John Wiley & Sons, Inc. Published 2017 by John Wiley & Sons, Inc.
Companion website: www.wiley.com/go/hubar/radiology

Protective apron

Protective covering to shield a patient from *scatter radiation* ☢☢ comes in many forms. The method of choice to date has been the protective apron (Fig. G1). The US Environmental Protection Agency (EPA) has designated *lead* as a hazardous material. Although the term *lead apron* is commonly used to describe the standard apron that is draped on a patient prior to x-ray exposure, many companies today manufacture lead-equivalent aprons (i.e. lead-free). Regarding intraoral procedures, assuming that one adheres to the guidelines outlined by the NCRP and ADA, there is no need to use a protective apron on adult patients due to the minute amount of scatter radiation outside of the field of interest. These guidelines require the use of rectangular collimation with either a digital receptor or f-speed film. The NCRP guidelines also state that pediatric patients are not simply small adult patients and operators should take extra care to reduce children's exposure to radiation. The thyroid gland in children sits higher in the neck and will therefore be automatically exposed to more radiation than in an adult. As a result, the NCRP recommends that protective aprons with *thyroid collars* ☢☢ should always be used on pediatric patients unless it interferes with imaging the needed anatomy. For extraoral imaging procedures such as panoramic projections, a double-sided protective apron without a thyroid collar should be used (Fig. G2). In this situation a thyroid collar would obscure anatomic structures that are relevant to the patient's oral examination.

Note: Do not fold the protective apron when not in use. It is best to either hang the apron upright or leave it lying flat and unfolded.

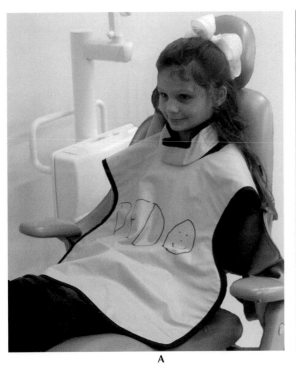
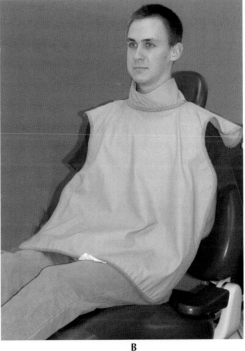

A   B

Fig. G1 A. Child protective apron with thyroid collar for intraoral imaging. B. Adult protective apron with thyroid collar for intraoral imaging.

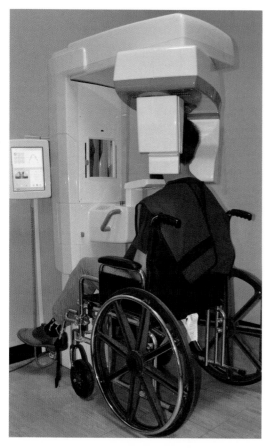

Fig. G2 Double-sided (i.e. front and back) protective apron *without thyroid collar* for extraoral imaging.

Repeated folding of the apron will lead to cracking of the inner lining and it will become less effective at blocking x rays. The NCRP also recommends a visual examination of protective aprons monthly for damage.

Collimation

The radiation produced within the x-ray tubehead exits as a divergent beam. The US government requires manufacturers of intraoral x-ray equipment to limit the size of the x-ray beam to be no more than 2.75 inches (7 cm) in diameter. The open-ended plastic attachment on the

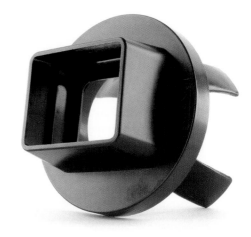

Fig. G3 Rinn® universal collimator which converts a round PID to a rectangular collimated PID to restrict the size of the x-ray beam to approximate the size of the image receptor.

x-ray tubehead is referred to as a *PID* ☢. A PID has historically been referred to as a *cone*. The open end of the PID is aligned closely to the patient's face prior to taking an exposure. A PID may be interchangeable on some intraoral tubeheads. Limiting the size of the beam reduces unnecessary exposure to the areas outside of the desired field. A means to further reduce the conventional round beam size is to use a rectangular-shaped beam that more closely matches the size of the imaging receptor (Figs G3, G4, G5 and G6). The NCRP guidelines state that rectangular collimation of the beam shall be used routinely for periapical and bitewing images and should be used for occlusal images when possible. In addition, rectangular collimation shall be used with hand-held devices when possible. If a rectangular PID is not already attached to the x-ray tubehead, a rectangular-shaped beam can still be accomplished by any one of the following solutions: (i) detaching the existing round PID and replacing it with a rectangular PID; (ii) a secondary rectangular collimator can be attached to the open end of the round PID; and (iii) a rectangular collimator can be attached

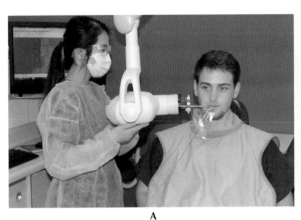

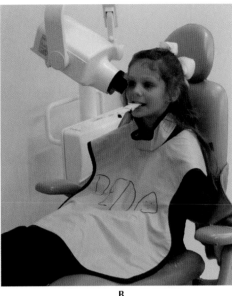

Fig. G4 A. Rectangular collimation with XCP-ORA® positioning system. B. Rectangular collimation with a Snap-A-Ray® DS (without an alignment ring).

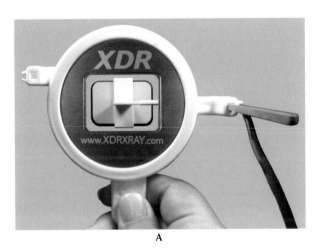

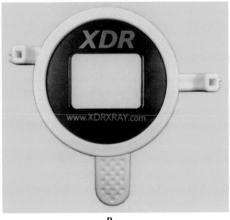

Fig. G5 XDR-ALARA® rectangular collimators.

directly to the receptor holder. For cephalometric images, the x-ray unit shall provide for appropriate collimation of the beam to the area of clinical interest. This will prevent unnecessary exposure to hard and soft tissues outside the area of interest.

Filtration

X-ray tubes simultaneously generate x rays of varying energies. The purpose of x-ray filtration is to absorb the weaker, low energy x rays that may not be powerful enough to penetrate

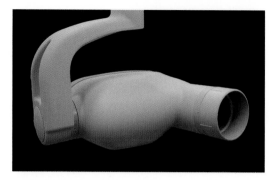

Fig. G6 Round PID collimation.

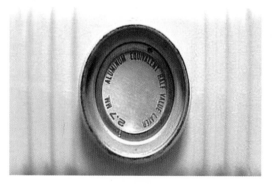

Fig. G7 Aluminum filter integrated into the body of the x-ray tubehead.

through a patient's soft tissue. Filtering out these low energy x-ray photons reduces the total absorbed dose to the patient and will not compromise the final diagnosis. X-ray filters typically made of aluminum are inherently built into conventional dental x-ray units (Fig. G7). In the United States, manufacture of x-ray equipment is regulated by the Food and Drug Administration (FDA) and consequently x-ray filtration should not be a concern for clinicians.

Digital versus analog

The world's first digital dental intraoral system was introduced in 1987 by the French company Trophie Radiologie; it was called *RadioVisio-Graphy*. Today, many different manufacturers

produce dental digital receptors. Digital receptors have significantly reduced the total dose of radiation required to produce diagnostic images that are comparable to the prior standard image receptor, dental x-ray film. Looking back to the earliest intraoral x-ray images back in 1896, exposure times were upwards of 25 min in length. Today's dental exposure time is typically only a fraction of a second in length, thereby dramatically reducing a patient's overall exposure to radiation compared with the historical doses that many patients received during the early days of dental radiology. The recent transition from x-ray film to a digital receptor is not as dramatic a dose reduction as that of the cumulative advances that occurred with film over the decades, but it has definitely contributed to further dose reduction to the patient.

Exposure settings

Radiation exposure dose to a patient is directly controlled by the operator's selection of kilovolt peak (kVp), milliamperage (mA) and exposure time. However, optimum settings are subjective; one size does not fit all here. Each dentist has their own image quality preferences. In addition, an x-ray unit's radiation output will vary according to the age of the unit, manufacturer's specs, etc. In this regard, government inspectors will periodically inspect each dental office's x-ray equipment to ensure that their equipment is operating according to the manufacturer's guidelines. Improper functioning x-ray equipment may result in unnecessary additional radiation exposure to the patient.

Operator technique

An operator's technique is critical in producing diagnostic images with minimal distortion, missed apices, etc. Undiagnostic images will require re-exposure of the patient. Intraoral instrumentation for holding the receptor and aligning the PID do not guarantee acquisition of diagnostic images, they simply aid the patient and the operator in the attempt to acquire a good diagnostic image. Similarly, the operator's proper exposure setting selection and patient positioning in an extraoral unit will reduce the number of unnecessary retakes.

2. RADIATION PROTECTION: OFFICE PERSONNEL

The NCRP requires that the construction and design of a dental office must include safety features to protect all personnel working with or near x-ray equipment. In addition, the owner of a dental practice must protect the front-end personnel such as receptionists and those individuals working in adjacent offices to reduce their exposure to dental x radiation.

The NCRP x-ray protection guidelines for dental offices are as follows:

- *The dentist (or, in some facilities, the designated radiation safety officer) shall establish a radiation protection program. The dentist shall seek guidance of a qualified expert.*
- *The qualified expert should provide guidance for the dentist or facility engineer in the layout and shielding design of new or renovated dental facilities and when equipment is installed that will significantly increase the air* kerma ☢ *[kinetic energy released per unit mass] incident in walls, floors and ceilings.*
- *New dental facilities shall be designed such that no individual member of the public will receive an effective dose in excess of 1 mSv annually.*
- *The qualified expert should perform a pre-installation radiation shielding design and plan review to determine the proper location and composition of barriers used to ensure radiation protection in new or extensively remodeled facilities and when equipment is installed that will significantly increase the air kerma incident in walls, floors and ceilings.*
- *Shielding design for new offices for planned fixed x-ray equipment installations shall provide protective barriers for the operator. The barriers shall be constructed*

so operators can maintain visual contact and communication with patients throughout the procedures.
- *The exposure switch should be mounted behind the protective barrier such that the operator must remain behind the barrier during the exposure (Fig. G8).*
- *Adequacy of shielding shall be determined by the qualified expert whenever workload increases by a factor of two or more from initial design criteria.*
- *In the absence of a barrier in an existing facility, the operator shall remain at least two meters, but preferably three meters from the x-ray tubehead during exposure. If the two meter distance cannot be maintained, then a barrier shall be provided. This recommendation does not apply to hand-held units with integral shielding.*
- *The qualified expert should perform a post-installation radiation protection survey to assure that radiation exposure levels in nearby public and controlled areas are ALARA and below the level limits established by the state and other local agencies with jurisdiction.*
- *The qualified expert should assess each facility individually and document the recommended shielding in a written report.*
- *The qualified expert should consider the cumulative radiation exposures resulting from representative workloads*

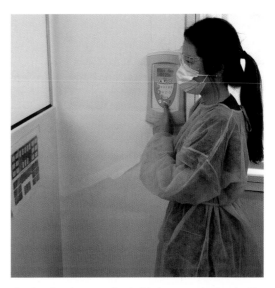

Fig. G8 Operator standing behind a protective barrier (the lower portion is a lead shield and the upper portion is made of leaded glass) during radiation exposure of a patient.

in each modality when designing radiation shielding for rooms in which there are multiple x-ray machines.

- *A qualified expert shall evaluate x-ray equipment to ensure that it is in compliance with applicable laws and regulations.*
- *All new dental x-ray installations shall have [a] radiation protection survey and equipment performance evaluation carried out by or under the direction of a qualified expert.*
- *For new or relocated equipment, the facilities shall provide personal dosimeters for at least one year in order to determine and document the doses to personnel.*
- *Equipment performance evaluations shall be performed at regular intervals thereafter, preferably at intervals not to exceed four years for facilities only with intraoral, panoramic or cephalometric units. Facilities with CBCT units shall be evaluated every one to two years.*

Source: National Council on Radiation Protection and Measurement (2017)

Practitioners must comply if they want to eliminate or at least reduce their risk of potential liability.

Additional methods to protect an operator from occupational exposure to radiation include the following:

1. If assistance is required for a child or a handicapped patient to stabilize the receptor instrument, non-occupationally exposed persons (preferably a member of the patient's family) should be asked to assist so that the operator can stand outside the operatory. Offering the volunteer a protective apron may reduce any apprehension the individual might have about being exposed alongside the patient. The rationale for substituting a surrogate is because this individual will be exposed to a minimum of radiation exposure possibly this one occasion, while the operator may be required to repeat this procedure on numerous different patients and thereby receive far greater cumulative levels of radiation exposure.

2. When a protective barrier is unavailable, the operator should stand at least 2 m from the x-ray tubehead and between 90° and 135° from the direction of the primary x-ray beam. Standing distance measured from the x-ray source incorporates the *inverse square law* ☢ which allows for additional dissipation of the x rays. This standing position also utilizes the patient's body as a barrier for absorbing some of the scattered x rays (Fig. G9).

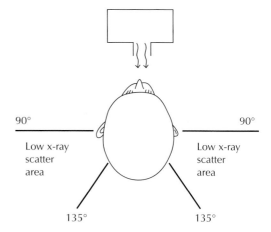

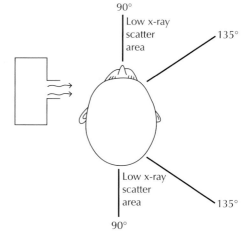

Fig. G9 Illustration demonstrating the safest position for the operator to stand when there is no protective barrier and the operator is within 2 m of the patient.

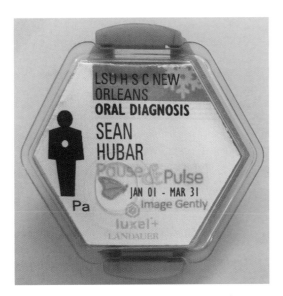

Fig. G10 Radiation dosimeter badge (clip-on style).

The monitoring of radiation exposure to personnel in a dental office is typically accomplished through the use of an individual *radiation dosimetry badge* ☢ (Fig. G10). The NCRP guidelines (2017) state that "Provision of personal dosimeters for external exposure measurement should be considered for workers who are likely to receive an annual effective dose in excess of 1 mSv. Personal dosimeters shall be provided for declared pregnant occupationally-exposed personnel" (see Section P).

How much occupational radiation exposure is permitted?

Both the NCRP and the International Commission on Radiological Protection (ICRP) have published guidelines for occupational and non-occupational dose limits. The NCRP and ICRP state that occupational workers should not be exposed to more than 50 millisieverts (mSv) per year, referred to as *maximum permissible dose (MPD)* ☢. The calculated value of an individual's total lifetime occupational effective dose shall be limited to 10 mSv multiplied by the age of that individual. For example, a total lifetime occupational exposure for a 25-year-old worker is 25 × 10 = 250 mSv. In reality, if a proper safety protocol is adhered to in a dental office, occupational doses should fall well below the MPD. However, if the operator's exposure level exceeds the permitted annual level, the operator would be temporarily prohibited from working around x-ray equipment until the accumulated dose fell below the level permitted based on the 50 mSv/year calculation.

Note: There is no MPD for patients because the radiation exposure that healthcare professionals deliver is deemed to be beneficial for the patient in either a diagnostic or a therapeutic capacity. Obviously, keeping the patient exposure dose to a minimum should be a primary objective.

Patient Selection Criteria

The dentist must weigh the benefits of taking dental radiographs against the risk of exposing a patient to x rays, the effects of which accumulate from multiple sources over time. The dentist, knowing the patient's health history and vulnerability to oral disease, is in the best position to make this judgment in the interest of each patient. For this reason, the guidelines are intended to serve as a resource for the practitioner and are not intended as standards of care, requirements or regulations.

Source: American Dental Association Council on Scientific Affairs (2006)

The ADA guidelines quoted above differentiate between symptomatic and asymptomatic patients. For symptomatic patients, a radiographic examination should be limited to images required for diagnosis and planned treatment of current disease. In a radiographic examination of asymptomatic patients such as new patients or returning patients, the practitioner should adhere to published selection criteria. The operative word in the ADA statement is "guidelines." All healthcare providers must use their good judgment when prescribing x-ray images as they are not limited to or prohibited from requesting any x-ray image if it may benefit the patient's care (see Appendix 1).

The ADA guidelines for prescribing images vary amongst different demographic groups, although this is not to say that a particular health concern can only occur in a specific group. Historically there are patterns that warrant modifying imaging protocol to accommodate these variations. As mentioned earlier, the dental practitioner has the authority to request whatever x-ray images are deemed necessary for a thorough diagnosis of the patient. Pre-existing dental x-ray images taken at other dental offices should also be obtained whenever possible before prescribing new x-ray procedures. A chronological sequence of dental images can be very useful for documenting both developmental and pathological changes to the oral cavity. All patients are entitled to copies of dental images and may request them from their current or former dentist(s). Additional fees may be incurred by the patient for producing copies of x-ray images. It is at the discretion of each dental practitioner to decide whether to charge or waive any fees for this service. All dental practitioners should keep permanent records of all x-ray images for all current and former patients. Why? This is because a dentist may be called upon to produce x-ray images to assist in the postmortem forensic identification of an individual or possibly the dentist may be at the center of a legal dispute arising from a disgruntled patient who has filed a lawsuit. Pre- and post-treatment x-ray images can be vital in the dentist's legal defense for disproving false claims about performing unnecessary or poor quality dental treatment.

What about pregnant patients? To be safe, it is always best to avoid exposing the mother to any x-ray images during the entire term of her pregnancy. The risks to the developing fetus are known to be minimal but the dentist does not want to be indicted afterwards by the mother as being the cause of a child's unforeseen birth defect. However, treating the mother's dental problem is also essential to the health of the developing baby. If the mother is experiencing undue stress or has an untreated dental infection, more harm could result to the baby than by exposing a few intraoral x-ray images and properly treating the oral problem. The author recommends that the dentist expose the minimum number of x-ray images necessary to treat the current problem and to take all precautions to reduce the radiation exposure to the patient. Additional protection for the fetus is made possible by placing a full-length protective apron on the patient. This will absorb 99.9% of the stray x rays that might reach the mother's abdominal region. Of course, elective treatment should be postponed until after birth of the child.

Film versus Digital Imaging

Film

X rays were first discovered in 1895. At that time emulsion-coated glass plates were used to record both photographic and x-ray images. The first commercial roll of photographic film was introduced in 1899 by the Eastman Kodak Company. However, the transition to using flexible film rather than glass plates to record x-ray images did not occur until the 1910s. Once flexible x-ray film was introduced, it was repeatedly improved over the years until its use began to decline with the introduction of digital imaging beginning in the 1980s. The last significant advancement in x-ray film was back in the year 2000 when Kodak introduced "Insight" intraoral film. From the earliest days of x rays, when a 20 min exposure to radiation may have been required to produce an x-ray image, the last incarnation of intraoral film reduced the patient exposure time to seconds.

Two categories of dental x-ray film are *non-screen* and *screen film*. Intraoral x-ray film is a *non-screen* film type, also referred to as a direct exposure film. It is composed of a flexible piece of transparent cellulose acetate which acts as the base to support an emulsion that is coated on both the front and the back sides. This emulsion consists of silver halide crystals suspended in a thin layer of gelatin. To protect the soft gelatin from incurring damage from mishandling, it is manufactured with a protective coating applied over it. X-ray film is not only sensitive to x rays but also to white light sources. Consequently, intraoral x-ray film is individually prepackaged in a sealed, lightproof packet. This protective packet prevents the film from being exposed to white light and it also prevents the patient's saliva from contaminating the film's emulsion. Within each intraoral film packet there is also a thin sheet of lead foil located behind the film and a piece of black paper. The lead foil serves two functions:

1. It provides additional protection to the patient by absorbing some of the incoming and scattered x rays. Some x rays can ricochet off the teeth and bones behind the film packet and could expose the film from the backside. These scattered x rays would contribute to degrading the quality of the final image. This effect is referred to as *film fog*. The lead foil blocks these back-scattered x rays and thereby reduces film fog.

Fundamentals of Oral and Maxillofacial Radiology, First Edition. J. Sean Hubar.
© 2017 John Wiley & Sons, Inc. Published 2017 by John Wiley & Sons, Inc.
Companion website: www.wiley.com/go/hubar/radiology

2. Embossed upon each piece of lead foil is a geometric pattern that each manufacturer selects (e.g. honeycomb). If the operator erred and placed the film packet reversed in the patient's mouth and exposed it, the foil's embossed pattern would now be visible on the final image and this would alert the dentist that the image must be reversed to properly orientate the patient's dentition. Failure to do so could lead to performing unnecessary dental treatment on healthy teeth and leaving untreated diseased teeth.

Extraoral x-ray film is classified as a *screen film*. As the term *extraoral* infers, these films are positioned outside of the patient's mouth during an x-ray exposure. This category of film is always sandwiched between two *intensifying screens* within a light-tight film cassette. An intensifying screen's composition includes layers of phosphor crystals. When a phosphor crystal in the screen is hit by an x-ray photon, it fluoresces. This fluorescent light diverges and simultaneously exposes multiple halide crystals in the film. As a result, intensifying screens help to reduce the total amount of radiation exposure to the patient but they also produce an image with poorer *image resolution* ☢ compared with a non-screen film image. Consequently, non-screen intraoral films are better for diagnosing small lesions like caries where finer detail is required. Intensifying screens are not used with intraoral films.

Whether an operator uses a screen or a non-screen film, the exposed x-ray film needs to be chemically processed before a dental image will be visible to our eyes. The hidden image on an unprocessed x-ray film is referred to as a *latent image*. Processing can either be performed manually by the operator or with a *film processor* ☢, where the film is automatically drawn through the solutions. Either way, the film must be processed in a dark environment to avoid extraneous exposure to white light. Chemical processing of a dental film consists of first submerging each film into a developing solution for a specified time, then the films are submersed in a fixer solution for a set length of time and finally each film is washed in water. The function of the developer solution is to precipitate the silver atoms within the emulsion, the fixer serves to remove the unaffected crystals and water removes all traces of the chemical solutions. The precipitated silver appears black on the image. A film accidentally exposed to white light will turn totally black during processing. Proponents of x-ray film generally claim that dental images acquired on x-ray film are still superior to digital receptor images.

Digital imaging

In 1987, the first digital image receptor was introduced for intraoral imaging. Since that time, digital imaging has gradually become the new standard for acquiring and viewing of dental images.

Direct digital imaging refers to directly capturing a latent image onto an appropriate receptor. Currently, there are two different technologies of intraoral digital systems. One system incorporates solid state electronics that use either *CCD* ☢ (charge coupled device) or *CMOS* ☢ (complementary metal oxide semiconductor) technology (Fig. I1). Both the CMOS and CCD receptors typically are wired directly to a

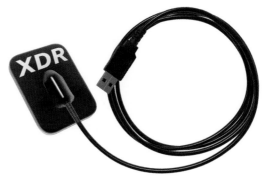

Fig. I1 Direct digital receptor. (Source: Courtesy of Adam Chen, XDR Radiology.)

computer. However, some manufacturers have introduced a modified direct system that uses a Wi-Fi signal to transmit the data from the receptor directly to the computer rather than via a physical wire. in either wired or Wi-Fi signal transmission, both receptor designs directly send the image to a computer. The alternative digital receptor technology uses *photostimulable phosphor plates (PSP plates)* (Fig. I2). A phosphor coating is deposited onto a thin, flexible piece of polyester acetate. The x-ray image is captured and stored as a *latent image* in the phosphor coating. Each manufacturer of PSP plates produces a specific scanner to digitize the acquired latent images.

Indirect digital imaging refers to the conversion of the latent analog image captured on a PSP plate into a digital image. Once the PSP plate has been scanned, the image can be erased by exposing the PSP plate to a room-intensity white light. A PSP plate can be erased and re-exposed multiple times. Operator care should

be taken not to scratch or bend the PSP plate so as to prolong its functional life. The flexibility and thinness of the PSP plate makes it much more patient friendly. Unlike the limited selection of solid-state digital receptor sizes, PSP plates come in several different sizes. PSP plate image quality is comparable to solid-state digital images but the added time and steps involved to visualize the digital image make it unappealing to many practitioners at this time. On the flip side, the cost for each intraoral PSP plate is minimal. Typical cost ranges between twenty-five and thirty-five dollars per intraoral PSP plate compared to thousands of dollars for a single solid-state receptor.

Dental equipment manufacturers may offer three sizes (0, 1 and 2) of solid-state intraoral digital receptors. Digital receptor sizes closely match intraoral film sizes. Numerically, the higher the receptor number, the larger is the physical area that is captured in the image. Of the three different choices, size 2 acquires the largest area while

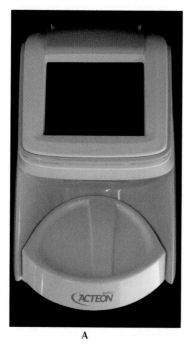

A

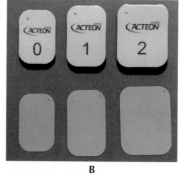

B

Fig. I2 A. PSP plate scanner. B. PSP plates and pouches: sizes 0, 1 and 2.

0 acquires the smallest area. Most operators use size 2 for all posterior periapical views and also for bitewing images, while size 1 is used for anterior periapical views. Size 0 is ideal for children whose smaller mouths accommodate it much better. This will be discussed further in Section L on intraoral techniques. Solid-state intraoral receptors are currently not made larger than a size 2. Limited demand for larger intraoral images such as occlusal views and the high price to manufacture larger size solid-state receptors are the obvious reasons why they are not available today. PSP plates, because of their modest prices, are available in larger sizes.

Advantages of digital x-ray imaging

Digital imaging has always been marketed as being a significant time saver in comparison to using dental x-ray film. This is somewhat true. It is accurate that a solid-state digital receptor can process an image in mere seconds, but PSP plates require added time because the operator must scan each PSP plate individually. In addition, each plate must "blanked" to reuse it and then repackaged. Consequently, operational time savings are not as pronounced as may be expected using PSP systems.

Manufacturers also cite dose reduction to the patient as a significant benefit when using digital imaging systems compared with dental x-ray film. Historically, the first dental exposures were upwards of 25 min in length. Today, intraoral images using digital receptors typically utilize exposure times in mere thousandths of a second. To be fair, however, the latest intraoral dental x-ray film has reduced exposure times to a second in length, being only slightly more than a digital exposure setting. Manufacturers' claims of upwards of a 75% reduction in exposure time compared with using film in reality often translates into a mere fraction of a second reduction per exposure.

Unlike dental x-ray film, where "what you see is what you get," digital x-ray images, like digital photographs, can be easily altered to enhance them. Imaging software typically permits modifying image *brightness* ♠♠, *contrast* ♠♠ and *image resolution* ♠♠. As a consequence, a subdiagnostic digital image may be improved just enough that it may negate the need for a retake which would expose the patient to additional radiation. This applies to both solid-state and PSP plate receptors. In addition, combining an x-ray image with a clinical photograph on a screen offers the dental professional a powerful tool to educate patients. Viewing both images together allows the dentist to demonstrate the patient's specific dental problems and the proposed treatment options. Digital imaging technology facilitates transmission of dental images to fellow colleagues for consultation purposes or for the submission of images to dental insurance companies for pre-authorization of proposed treatment plans.

Patients may request copies of their x-ray images for a variety of reasons, such as they are relocating to another city and will be treated by a new dentist. Previously, with only x-ray film available, it was much more cumbersome to duplicate radiographs, especially since dentists have always been advised to keep the *original* radiographs and only supply copies to the patient and insurance companies. In the event a dentist is called to a court of law, original x-ray images are critical for the dentist's defense. It is important to mention that patients are legally entitled to copies, in any format, of all their x-ray images. The simple reason is that a patient should not have to be exposed to additional radiation simply because a dentist opted not to release the existing radiographs to the patient. However, it is up to the discretion of every dentist to decide whether or not to charge a duplication fee for providing this service to the patient.

Disadvantages of digital imaging

An obvious disadvantage of a solid-state intraoral receptor is its physical bulk. These receptors are typically several millimeters thick and are constructed with a rigid metal housing. Consequently, solid-state receptors may not be well tolerated by some patients and the operator may at times be unable to expose any intraoral images. However, most patients do cooperate and merely complain about the discomfort when solid-state receptors are used. In contrast, PSP plates, being very thin and flexible, often are better tolerated by patients. For this reason, PSP plates are generally considered more suitable for children whose reduced tolerance levels and smaller oral cavities further complicate positioning any type of intraoral receptor.

For proper infection control, plastic *protective barriers* ♣ are used to cover all varieties of intraoral image receptors. A solid-state receptor typically is inserted into a disposable protective sleeve, while a PSP plate typically is sealed in a single use plastic envelope. The edges and seams of the plastic barrier cover frequently irritate patients' soft tissues and as a consequence may initiate a pharyngeal spasm (i.e. gag reflex). The discomfort from the barrier cover is often described by patients as either "scratching" or "tickling" (see Fig. O2).

Dentists often ignore the importance of the monitor. The resolution of the monitor has a profound effect on the diagnostic quality of digital images, particularly when the images are enlarged. Viewing x-ray images on a lower resolution monitor in a brightly lit environment will significantly diminish the observer's ability to detect pathology. Consequently, a dentist should invest in a higher quality viewing monitor and locate it in a room with subdued lighting to improve diagnostic performance.

There is a high financial cost of using digital imaging. Each solid-state receptor is priced in the thousands of dollars and they are particularly vulnerable to mishandling. Compounding the initial cost outlay for the receptor(s), there may be a substantial annual cost for an insurance warranty for unforeseen damages unless one wishes to fully assume the repair costs,

which could also be in the thousands of dollars. In contrast, PSP plates themselves are very inexpensive. However, the PSP plates have a very limited lifespan, partly as a consequence of being prone to scratches, bends, etc. Even properly handled PSP plates will still need to be replaced regularly. More significant however is the initial cost of the PSP plate scanner. In the end, PSP plate and solid-state receptor systems are comparable in overall cost.

Imaging software

Today, x-ray manufacturers universally utilize the *DICOM* standard. DICOM is an abbreviation for **D**igital **I**maging and **Com**munication in **M**edicine. DICOM allows for exchanging files between different manufacturers' hardware and, more importantly, DICOM files enhance security. Attached to every image is the patient's identification which cannot be separated from the image. Consequently, digital images allow for easy transfer of patient x-ray records from one office to another or submission of digital images to insurance companies for work authorization and reimbursement.

Image enhancement

As with digital photographs, less than perfect digital x-ray images may be software enhanced to make them more diagnostically useful. Imaging software typically allows modification of contrast, brightness and resolution. The density of an x-ray film or a digital image always refers to its degree of darkness. If the captured image is too dark (i.e. overexposed) or too light (i.e. underexposed), modifying the image may be valuable in salvaging it. Filtration tools can alter the *sharpness* ♣ of an image. Filtering images is a personal preference. Some observers prefer sharper images to better delineate, for example, dental caries or bone levels, others may not. Other common enhancement tools include colorization and contrast reversal. The colorization feature converts the different shades of gray in an image to individual distinctive colors which may be useful for patient education. Reversing the contrast turns a positive image into a negative image. In this manner what appears black on the untouched image becomes white and vice versa. Neither this function, nor colorization, upgrades the diagnostic information on an image. They merely alter the visual perception of the image for the observer. Personal preference dictates their usefulness.

Image measurement

Imaging software programs incorporate a measurement tool. This can be used for determining tooth length, thicknesses, tooth spacing, etc. However, be aware that the software cannot account for technique (i.e. angulation) errors in the positioning of the receptor in the oral cavity. Consequently, elongation and foreshortening of the image will not be corrected by the software and as a result the measurements derived are not completely accurate.

In summary, software enhancement features are very useful. Different observers may have different visual preferences and therefore wish to alter the viewing ability of the image to suit their particular needs. This is not possible with x-ray film without exposing additional images. However, software alone may not be enough to eliminate retakes and, as a result of DICOM standards, image enhancements made to the original image are not permanent. This is critical in legal proceedings. Should a dentist be involved in a dispute with a patient and the matter went to court, the original unaltered digital images could be critical in determining the outcome of the case.

What do Dental X-ray Images Reveal?

Upon the discovery of x rays, it immediately occurred to those in the dental field that they would be an invaluable tool for observing inside the jaws and teeth. Modern x-ray equipment allows the operator to expose various types of dental images in the hope of improving a patient's overall oral health. Two- and three-dimensional intraoral and extraoral images are routinely used in treatment planning procedures involving endodontics, implants, oral pathology, oral surgery, orthodontics, pediatric dentistry, periodontics and prosthodontics.

X-ray images are beneficial for the detection of:

1. Alterations to the dentition
2. Periodontal disease
3. Growth and development
4. Alterations to the periapical tissues
5. Osseous pathology
6. Temporomandibular joint disorder
7. Implant assessment (pre- and post-placement)
8. Identification of a foreign body

Alterations to the dentition

Caries

Radiologically, enamel and dentin are differentiated based upon their individual mineral content (i.e. *hydroxyapatite* ♣). Enamel is over 90% mineralized by weight while dentin is approximately 65% mineralized. Demineralization of enamel and dentin is referred to as *dental caries*. It results from acid production by *Streptococcus* bacteria that are directly attached to one or more surfaces of a tooth. Demineralization of the tooth structure allows greater numbers of x-ray photons to penetrate through to the image receptor. Thus dental caries typically appear radiolucent on dental images. However, current digital receptors are not sensitive enough to detect less than 40% demineralization. This means that the percentage of demineralization has to exceed this threshold level before an individual is able to visualize and differentiate caries from normal tooth structure on a dental image. As a result, clinical caries will always be greater than the radiographic

Fundamentals of Oral and Maxillofacial Radiology, First Edition. J. Sean Hubar.
© 2017 John Wiley & Sons, Inc. Published 2017 by John Wiley & Sons, Inc.
Companion website: www.wiley.com/go/hubar/radiology

appearance of caries. This fact is critical to the clinician who is restoring a tooth with a deep carious lesion. Bitewing dental images are particularly beneficial for detecting interproximal caries. Caries limited to the occlusal surface are often more difficult to diagnose radiologically because of the sheer bulk of enamel surrounding the caries which can obscure the occlusal demineralization (see Section V).

Location of teeth

Dental images are very useful for localizing the positions of both erupted and unerupted teeth, visualizing tooth to tooth relationships and tooth to anatomic structures relationships. This information is essential for orthodontic and oral surgical treatment planning procedures. Teeth that are not in their proper sequential position are referred to as ectopic, transpositioned or translocated teeth.

Number of teeth

Unerupted teeth or the presence of *supernumerary* ☢ teeth can be easily observed on x-ray images. Clinically, a missing tooth might simply be due to the young developmental age of the patient or possibly the result of being *impacted* ☢. Both situations can be diagnosed with x-ray images. Supernumerary teeth may be single or multiple in number, unilateral or bilateral and in one or both jaws.

Shape of teeth

Abnormal tooth shape is typically developmental in origin. It may be the result of a congenital anomaly, associated with childhood facial trauma, or due to a localized oral infection. Congenital disorders include amelogenesis imperfecta, dentinogenesis imperfecta, dentinal dysplasia, taurodontism, dens in dente, fusion and germination (see Section W).

Integrity of the dentition

Physical changes to the integrity of a tooth can frequently be visualized on dental images. Examples include enamel or dentin demineralization, crown or root fractures and root resorption. All of these conditions appear as varying degrees of radiolucency on an otherwise normal image of a tooth. Alternatively, conditions can arise where calcification can occur internally within the pulp chamber or externally on the crown or root surface such as the deposition of calculus. Those affected areas will appear more radiopaque on a dental image. Poorer resolution of extraoral images compared with intraoral images may limit the visualization of some of these dental conditions.

Periodontal disease

Dental images are extremely beneficial for assessing the supporting bone surrounding the teeth, for evaluating widening of the periodontal ligament space and for visualizing the presence of calculus which predisposes an individual to bone loss, furcation involvement, etc. Bone loss surrounding the teeth can be measured by comparing the existing height of the alveolar ridge to the cervical area of the erupted teeth. The height of the alveolar bone surrounding a tooth normally is approximately 1.5 mm from the cemento-enamel junction. Interproximal bone loss is possible either parallel to or angled to the cemento-enamel junction and is commonly referred to as either *horizontal* or *vertical bone loss* ☢.

Growth and development

Skeletal changes to the orofacial complex primarily occur from birth through late adolescence. X-ray images are vital for assessing growth development to consider the need for orthodontic treatment or orofacial surgery.

Conventional extraoral projections such as panoramic, cephalographic images can be used to monitor a patient's growth and progress of their treatment. In addition, advanced imaging such as CBCT can prove to be invaluable diagnostic tools in many cases.

Alterations to periapical tissues

Radiologic changes associated with the periapical tissues include widening of the periodontal ligament space, loss of the lamina dura and the presence of a radiopacity or radiolucency at the apex of a tooth. Infection, trauma or a metabolic disease may be the cause(s) for these osseous changes.

Osseous pathology

Factors contributing to osseous changes to the mandible and maxilla include congenital and metabolic diseases, trauma, infection and neoplasms. Number, location, density, shape, size, borders and changes to surrounding structures such as root resorption and tooth displacement are all necessary to determine a differential diagnosis. However, the final determination of a diagnosis often relies on a biopsy. Density can be altered to become more radiolucent or more radiopaque or to be a combination of both (i.e. mixed). Typically, an aberrant radiolucency within the jaws is indicative of a destructive process, a radiopacity is indicative of a calcifying process and a mixed radiolucent–radiopaque lesion can be either.

Temporomandibular joint disorder

Conventional extraoral projections such as a panoramic image have limited benefit when it comes to diagnosing osseous changes in the temporomandibular joint. CBCT imaging of the temporomandibular joint has become the standard of care for observing articular bony defects, flattening, osteophyte formation and sclerotic changes of the condyle. Imaging of the articular disk is not visible on x-ray images, however it can be identified with *magnetic resonance imaging (MRI)* ☢.

Implant assessment (pre- and post-placement)

X-ray images are invaluable both in pre-surgical planning and postoperative evaluation of implant placement. In particular, cross-sectional CBCT images assist pre-surgical treatment planning for assessing bone height, bone width and visualization of anatomic variations and anatomic structures such as the mandibular canal. Today many clinicians incorporate implant planning software in conjunction with CBCT imagery for determining the correct size and path of implant placement. Postoperative imaging frequently is also useful in assessing failing implants and to assist in determining causation of chronic postoperative pain.

Identification of a foreign body

A foreign body is any extraneous object that is introduced into the body. As a result, the size, shape and image density of a foreign body is variable. Generally, it will appear radiopaque on an x-ray image. The density of the radiopacity will vary depending upon its consistency (e.g. metal, plastic, glass). Localization of a foreign body can sometimes be easily accomplished with the *SLOB rule* ☢ using intraoral images. Foreign bodies include broken dental instruments, bullet fragments, tooth fragments and sialoliths.

K

Intraoral Imaging Techniques

Two fundamental intraoral techniques can be used independently or combined for positioning an image receptor: the *paralleling* and the *bisecting angle* techniques. In general, regardless of which technique the operator decides to utilize, the operator should first be familiar with basic oral anatomy. Basic knowledge of the number of roots for each tooth and the root configuration of multirooted teeth are essential to capture the entire apical region. Secondly, with only the crowns of erupted teeth visible to the operator, a mental visualization of the long axes of teeth is useful for accurate receptor placement. The long axis of a tooth is an imaginary line that extends lengthwise through the center of the tooth. The long axis will vary from tooth to tooth. A maxillary central incisor's root is inclined so that the long axis points toward the *bregma* ☢ of the skull, whereas the long axes of maxillary molars generally point toward a *mid-sagittal* ☢ line at the top of the skull.

The ADA requires that every patient must first be clinically examined by a dentist before any x-ray images are exposed. Patient selection criteria must be used to determine the number and type of images to be exposed. The old practice of routinely exposing a full mouth series on all patients does not apply today (see Appendix 1).

Conventional intraoral exams may incorporate a combination of periapical, bitewing and, occasionally, occlusal images. A *full mouth series* of images is designed to show every tooth in both the mandible and the maxilla. Generally speaking, a full mouth series may contain upwards of 21 individual images (Fig. K1). The final tally of images exposed will also vary depending upon the size of the receptors used. An operator may find it preferable to use a larger receptor and capture several teeth on a single image rather than exposing two images using a smaller receptor, thereby reducing the total number of images required. However, the advantage of capturing additional teeth on a single image often may be negated by the production of less diagnostic images. Separation of interproximal contacts along a curved dental arch requires continually varying the horizontal angulation. If the resultant image has overlapped contacts, it can partially or entirely obscure dental caries, fractures, etc. (see Section L).

A *periapical image* is defined as a projection that captures the entire length of one or more teeth, extending from the incisal or occlusal edge to the apex of each root and the surrounding tissues. Two millimeters of bone visible beyond the apex of a tooth is desirable for the observer to confidently rule out disorders such

Fundamentals of Oral and Maxillofacial Radiology, First Edition. J. Sean Hubar.
© 2017 John Wiley & Sons, Inc. Published 2017 by John Wiley & Sons, Inc.
Companion website: www.wiley.com/go/hubar/radiology

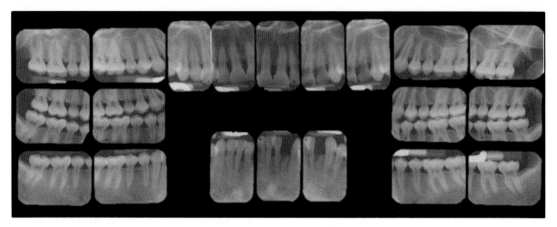

Fig. K1 Sample full mouth series of intraoral images.

as apical pathology. The term *periapical* image can also apply to edentulous regions of the mouth. Imaging edentulous areas where teeth previously were located is just as important as imaging dentulous regions. In fact, imaging edentulous regions may reveal unexpected pathology, supernumerary teeth, retained root tips, etc. An exception to this requirement would be if a current panoramic image already exists. In this situation, only undiagnostic or suspicious areas should be supplemented with higher resolution periapical images.

A *bitewing image* simultaneously shows the coronal portions of both the maxillary and the mandibular teeth. Ideally it will also show the height of the surrounding alveolar bone. However, if there has been significant bone loss, the crestal bone height may be absent from the image. The unique advantages of bitewing images include: (i) the visualization of open proximal contacts; and (ii) a more accurate representation of crestal bone height. In addition to revealing interproximal decay, open proximal contacts will reveal overfilled or underfilled restorations, recurrent decay, calculus deposits, etc.

An *occlusal image* reveals a bucco-lingual perspective that is not visible on either a peri-apical or a bitewing image. It is useful for observing expansion of cortical plates, isolating a foreign body, visualizing displacement of fractures, etc. It is also a particularly useful technique when patients have limited mouth opening and are unable to permit the placement of instrumentation for periapical images. The image receptor is placed between the occlusal surfaces of opposing arches and the patient is instructed to gently bite together to support the receptor in position. The PID is then aligned using either the paralleling or bisecting angle technique.

1. PARALLELING TECHNIQUE

The principles of the *paralleling technique* (aka long cone technique) requires that: (i) the long axis of the tooth and the image receptor are positioned parallel to one another; and (ii) the incoming x-ray beam must be directed perpendicular to both of them (Figs K2 and K3). If the operator follows these two principles, it will result in minimal image distortion. To properly maintain the receptor's intraoral position, the use of a receptor holding instrument is standard protocol. Manufacturers fabricate

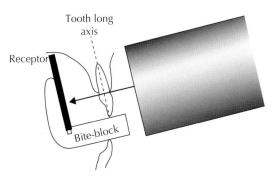

Fig. K2 Diagram showing the principles of the paralleling technique for all intraoral views. The image receptor is placed parallel to the long axis of the tooth and the x-ray beam is directed at a right angle to the receptor. A long x-ray source to image receptor distance of 30 cm is preferred.

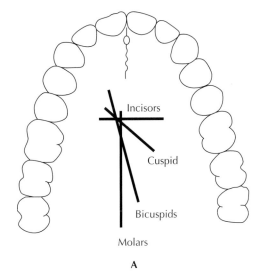

A

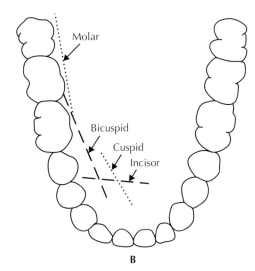

B

Fig. K3 A. Occlusal perspective showing the individual positions of the image receptor on the palatal side of the maxillary teeth for each periapical view. B. Occlusal perspective showing the individual positions of the image receptor on the lingual side of the mandibular teeth for each periapical view.

different styles of instrumentation for holding film, PSP plates and solid-state receptors. All of these devices are designed to stabilize the attached receptor. It is highly unlikely that a patient can maintain the receptor in its proper position using fingers alone for the entire length of the procedure. To achieve maximum stability, the operator should insert the instrument together with a receptor intraorally and then ask the patient to gently close their upper and lower teeth together for the duration of the image acquisition. A patient in this closed-mouth position is less likely to move compared with an open-mouth patient trying to maintain a constant position without using an instrument. Finally, to produce a beam of x rays that emanates from the end of a PID with minimal spatial divergence, a long *x-ray source* ☢ to receptor distance is required. The longer the distance from the source to the receptor, the greater will be the parallelism of the x-ray beam. X-ray parallelism produces less object magnification. However, there are practical limitations to the distance selected. A longer source to receptor distance requires a longer exposure time. It may also become physically difficult for the operator to align a longer PID in a space-constrained operatory. Typically, positioning the x-ray source 30 cm from the receptor is preferred.

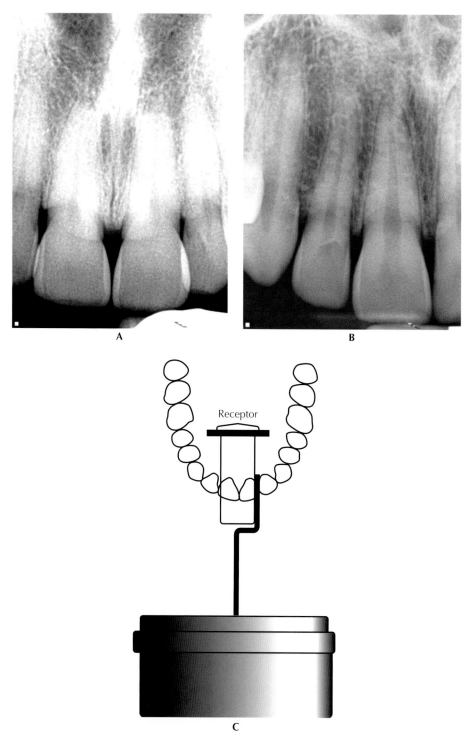

Fig. K4   A. Maxillary central incisors periapical view. B. Maxillary central and lateral incisors periapical view. C. Illustration demonstrating central incisors positioning of the receptor intraorally.

Maxillary incisors paralleling projection (Fig. K4)

Area of interest: Both the central and the lateral incisors.

Receptor size: No. 1 (preferable for ease of placement) or no. 2.

Position: The long dimension of the receptor is positioned *vertically*. The receptor should be rotated parallel to the labial surfaces of the central incisor and lateral incisor and set as far back palatally as possible. The posterior aspect of the oral cavity allows the receptor to be positioned higher in the palate to capture the apical regions of the teeth. An additional midline view of the two central incisors may be warranted to better visualize the interproximal surfaces of the two central incisors. If so, the receptor should be aligned parallel to the labial surfaces of the central incisors and set back as far posteriorly as possible.

Maxillary cuspid paralleling projection (Fig. K5)

Area of interest: Cuspid.

Receptor size: No. 2. The cuspid is generally the longest tooth in the mouth and as a result the smaller receptor may be too short to capture the entire length of the tooth.

Position: Regardless of which size receptor is used, the long dimension of the receptor must be attached *vertically*. Similar to the incisor view, the receptor must be positioned further palatally away from the cuspid. However, the horizontal angulation of the x-ray beam should be directed through the contact area between the cuspid and first bicuspid to minimize overlapping of these two teeth. Curvature of the maxillary arch will undoubtedly result in partial superimposition of the first bicuspid

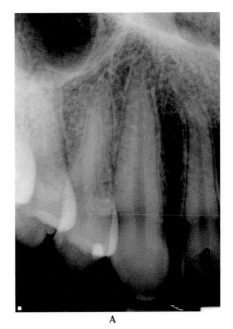

A

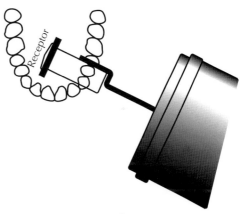

B

Fig. K5 A. Maxillary cuspid periapical view. B. Illustration demonstrating positioning of the receptor intraorally.

onto the distal surface of the cuspid. However, the distal contact of the cuspid ideally will be open and visible on one or both of the bicuspid bitewing view or the bicuspid periapical view.

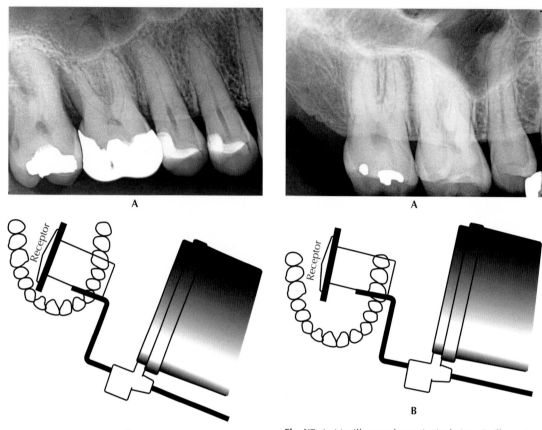

Fig. K6 A. Maxillary bicuspid periapical view. B. Illustration demonstrating positioning of the receptor intraorally.

Fig. K7 A. Maxillary molar periapical view. B. Illustration demonstrating positioning of the receptor intraorally.

Maxillary bicuspid paralleling projection (Fig. K6)

Area of interest: First and second bicuspids.

Receptor size: No. 2.

Position: For this projection, the long dimension of the receptor must be attached *horizontally*. Intraorally, the receptor should be aligned parallel to both the buccal surfaces and the long axes of the teeth. To achieve this, the operator will need to position the receptor towards the midline of the palate. This is the deepest area of the palatal vault and consequently will increase the likelihood of capturing the apices of the teeth on the image with minimal distortion of the teeth.

Maxillary molar paralleling projection (Fig. K7)

Area of interest: First, second and third molars.

Receptor size: No. 2.

Position: Similar to the bicuspid projection, the long dimension of the receptor must be positioned *horizontally*. Intraorally, the receptor should be aligned parallel to both the buccal surfaces and the long axes of the teeth. To achieve this, the operator will need to position the receptor towards the midline of the palate. This is the deepest area of the palatal vault and consequently will increase the likelihood of capturing the apices of the teeth on the image with minimal distortion of the teeth. The anterior aspect of the receptor should be positioned at approximately the middle of the second bicuspid tooth to ensure visualization of the mesial contact area of the first molar, and the posterior extent of the receptor ideally should extend to the maxillary tuberosity region. The receptor may not be large enough to capture the entire region desired in a single view. If a full mouth series of images is being taken, then the operator may decide that the bicuspid view already captured the first molar on it. Consequently, the operator can then position the receptor as far posteriorly as possible to capture the tuberosity region with only the second and third molars. To avoid unnecessary retakes, position the receptor initially in the bicuspid region and ask the patient to move the receptor as far posteriorly in their mouth as they can tolerate. After doing so, if the tuberosity region is still not captured on the image, the operator should resort to acquiring an extraoral image. A panoramic image would be the image of choice to see this region.

Mandibular incisor paralleling projection (Fig. K8)

Area of interest: Incisors.

Receptor size: No. 1 (preferable for ease of placement) or no. 2.

Position: The long dimension of the receptor is attached *vertically*. The instrument should be rotated so that the receptor is positioned parallel to the labial surfaces of the incisors and set beneath the patient's tongue. However, patient discomfort may prohibit proper seating of the receptor resulting in images with missed apices. In this region, as a result of short root lengths compared with the length of the receptor, positioning the receptor upon the dorsal surface of the tongue is permissible.

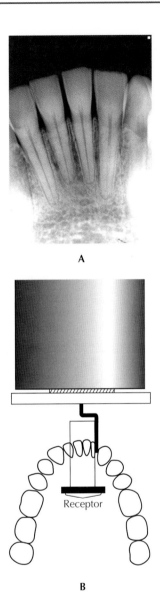

Fig. K8 A. Mandibular incisor view. B. Illustration demonstrating positioning of the receptor intraorally.

Additionally, the receptor should be positioned lingually back away from the labial surfaces of the teeth, which often alleviates patient discomfort and allows the individual to fully bite down on the instrument and thus capture the apices on the image.

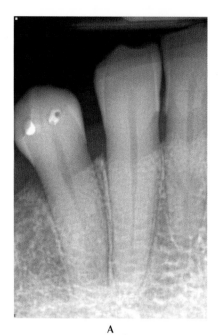

A

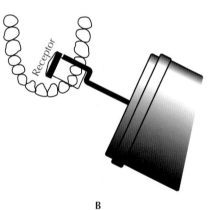

B

Fig. K9 A. Mandibular cuspid view. B. Illustration demonstrating positioning of the receptor intraorally.

Mandibular cuspid paralleling projection (Fig. K9)

Area of interest: Cuspid.

Receptor size: No. 2. The cuspid is generally the longest tooth in the mouth and as a result the smaller receptor may be too short to capture the entire length of the tooth. A larger receptor may be more appropriate to use in this situation.

Position: The long dimension of the receptor must be attached *vertically*. The receptor must be positioned lingually away from the cuspid. Similar to the mandibular incisors view, patient discomfort may prohibit proper seating of the receptor resulting in images with missed apices. Placement of the receptor on the dorsal surface of the tongue may help alleviate patient discomfort. It also allows the individual to fully bite down and thus capture the apex on the image. The horizontal angulation of the x-ray beam should be aimed through the contact area between the cuspid and first bicuspid to minimize overlapping of these two teeth. Constriction and curvature of the mandibular arch will undoubtedly result in some superimposition of the first bicuspid onto the distal surface of the cuspid. However, the distal contact of the cuspid ideally will be open and be visible on one or both of the bicuspid bitewing view or the bicuspid periapical view.

Mandibular bicuspid paralleling projection (Fig. K10)

Area of interest: First and second bicuspids.

Receptor size: No. 2.

Position: Unlike the anterior region of the mouth, the long dimension of the receptor must be attached *horizontally*. The receptor should be aligned parallel to both the buccal surfaces and the long axes of the teeth. It should not be placed onto the dorsal surface of the tongue because the patient's tongue may prevent the receptor from extending inferior enough to capture the periapical regions of the teeth. Consequently, the receptor must be positioned between the patient's tongue and next to the alveolar ridge, which may be quite uncomfortable for the patient. The mandibular bicuspid region tends to be the most tissue-sensitive region of the oral cavity. Patient discomfort and the cumbersome size of a solid-state receptor often prevent the operator from

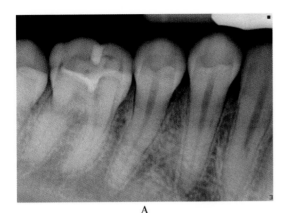

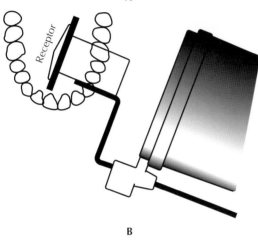

Fig. K10 A. Mandibular bicuspid view. B. Illustration demonstrating positioning of the receptor intraorally.

extending the receptor far enough anteriorly. This can result in cutting off the mesial portion of the first bicuspid from the image. Using a thinner and more flexible PSP plate will permit gentle bending of the receptor away from the sensitive mucosa. This should allow the operator to place a PSP plate more anteriorly and thereby capture the mesial surface of the first bicuspid on the image. However, care must be taken by the operator not to bend any PSP plate excessively as it may become permanently bent and reduce the PSP plate's usefulness for acquiring future images.

Mandibular molar paralleling projection (Fig. K11)

Area of interest: First, second and third molars.

Receptor size: No. 2.

Position: Similar to the bicuspid projection, the long dimension of the receptor must be positioned *horizontally*. Similar to the mandibular bicuspid view, the receptor should be aligned parallel to both the buccal surfaces and long axes of the teeth and should not be placed onto the dorsal surface of the tongue. Consequently, the receptor must be positioned between the patient's tongue and next to the alveolar ridge. It may not be quite as uncomfortable for a patient as it is for the bicuspid view as the receptor is positioned further from the very sensitive anterior mucosa. The anterior aspect of the receptor should be positioned at approximately the middle of the second bicuspid tooth to ensure visualization of the mesial contact area of the first molar, and the posterior extent of the receptor ideally extends to the retromolar region. Similar to the maxillary molar view, the receptor may not be large enough to capture this entire region in a single view. If a full mouth series of images is being exposed, then the operator may see that the bicuspid view has already captured the first molar on it. Consequently, the operator can then position the receptor further posteriorly to capture the retromolar region. Once again, to avoid unnecessary retakes, the operator should position the receptor initially in the bicuspid region and ask the patient, "Would you please move the receptor as far back in your mouth as you can?" Most patients will oblige and position the receptor even beyond your expectations. However, after requesting the patient to assist in the placement of the receptor, if the operator still determines that the region is not captured on the image, an extraoral projection such as a panoramic view should be prescribed to visualize the missing region.

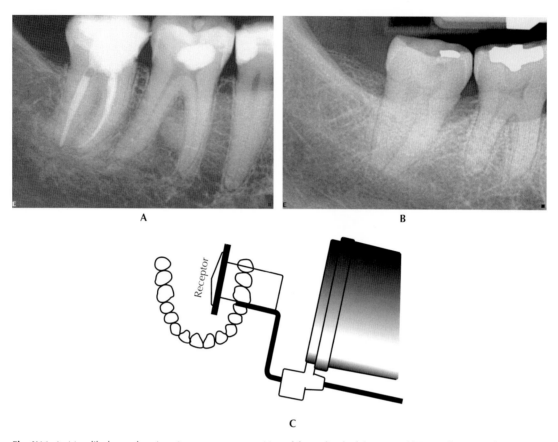

Fig. K11 A. Mandibular molar view. Image receptor positioned from distal of the second bicuspid posteriorly. B. Image receptor positioned as far posteriorly as a patient will physically tolerate to capture the retromolar region. The missing first molar will likely be visible on the bicuspid view. C. Illustration demonstrating positioning of the receptor intraorally.

2. BISECTING ANGLE TECHNIQUE

The *bisecting angle technique* ☢ is based on the rule of isometry, which makes this technique more complicated and difficult to perform without distortion of the x-ray image. The mathematical rule of *isometry* ☢ simply states that two triangles are equal when they share a common side. When applied to intraoral imaging, the long axis of a tooth and the plane of the receptor form two sides of a triangle. The operator must then visually bisect the angle of the two sides of the triangle and aim the x-ray beam perpendicular to this imaginary line (Fig. K12). The imaginary line is referred to as a bisector. Referring back to the principle of isometry, the bisector becomes the common side of two triangles.

Advantages of the bisecting angle technique include: (i) flexibility to position the receptor wherever the patient permits; (ii) no requirement for an instrument, although one may be used; and (iii) the use of either a short or a long PID.

Patients who have a hypersensitive gag reflex or a shallow palate, and young children whose mandibles are still growing, are not suitable for the paralleling technique; they can benefit from using the bisecting angle technqiue. Although exposure times are very short with both the bisecting and paralleling techniques, a short PID also permits using an even shorter exposure time, which can be critical for a patient with a hypersensitive gag response. Finally, operatory space limitations can complicate positioning a

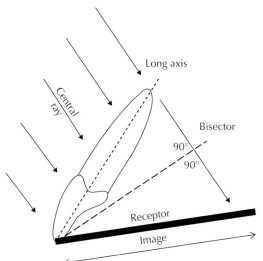

Fig. K12 Diagram showing the principles of the bisecting angle technique for all intraoral views. The x-ray beam is directed at right angles to a bisector determined by the position of the image receptor and long axis of the tooth.

long PID, which is mandatory for the paralleling technique. A short PID makes it easier for the operator to align it in a confined space.

Disadvantages of the bisecting angle technique include: (i) image distortion; (ii) the apices of the maxillary molars are obscured by the zygomatic arch; (iii) there is less detail of the root portion of the tooth compared with the coronal section; and (iv) a lack of standardization of PID alignment angles between patients. Incorrect vertical angulation (i.e. over- or underangulation) of the PID will distort the size of the image. *Overangulation* of the x-ray beam will *foreshorten* ☢ the image, while *underangulation* of the x-ray beam will *elongate* ☢ the image. In some situations the length of a tooth may be longer than the receptor's length and it cannot be fully imaged accurately. In this scenario, overangulation can be advantageous by intentionally making the tooth appear shorter so that it can be seen entirely in a single image. If rectangular collimation is being used, the operator may easily misalign the PID with the receptor and produce a cone-cut image. Of course, a cone-cut image may still occur with round collimation.

Maxillary incisor bisecting angle projection

Area of interest: Central and lateral incisors.

Receptor size: No. 1 (preferable for ease of placement) or no. 2.

Position: The receptor must be rotated so that its long dimension of the receptor is orientated *vertically*. The receptor should be centered behind the central and lateral incisors. The posterior edge of the receptor should be positioned as far palatally as possible while the anterior edge of the receptor should preferably extend 2 mm outward beyond the incisal edges. The mid-palatal and posterior aspect of the oral cavity allows the receptor to be positioned higher in the palate to capture the apical regions of the teeth. If an instrument is not used to hold the receptor in place, the patient's thumb may be used as the receptor holder. The back of the thumb should press the receptor up against the lingual side of the incisors. If a flexible PSP plate is used, gentle pressure of the thumb should be used to reduce bending of the receptor that would cause distortion of the image. The operator must then determine the correct vertical angulation of the PID by first visualizing the plane of the receptor and the long axes of the incisors. The angle that these two lines form must be visually bisected. The central ray of the PID should then be aimed perpendicular to this imaginary line with the lower edge of the PID extending beyond the edge of the receptor. An additional midline view of the two central incisors may be warranted on occasion to better visualize the mesial contacts of the two central incisors. If so, the receptor should be centrally aligned behind the lingual surfaces of the two central incisors.

Maxillary cuspid bisecting angle projection

Area of interest: Cuspid.

Receptor size: No. 2. The cuspid is generally the longest tooth in the mouth and as a result the smaller receptor may be too short to capture the entire length of the tooth. A larger receptor may be more appropriate to use in this situation.

Position: The receptor must be rotated so that its long dimension is orientated *vertically*. Similar to the incisor view, the receptor should be centered behind the cuspid and positioned across the mid-palatal line and as far posteriorly along the palate as possible. The horizontal angulation of the x-ray beam should be aimed through the contact area between the cuspid and first bicuspid to minimize overlapping of these two teeth. Curvature of the maxillary arch will undoubtedly result in partial superimposition of the first bicuspid onto the distal of the cuspid. However, the distal contact of the cuspid ideally will be open and visible on one or both of the bicuspid bitewing image or the bicuspid periapical image. The operator must then calculate the correct positive vertical angulation of the PID by first visualizing the plane of the receptor and the long axis of the cuspid. The angle that these two lines form must be bisected. The central ray of the PID should then be aimed perpendicular to this imaginary bisecting line with the lower edge of the PID extending beyond the edge of the receptor. At times an approximation of the correct vertical angle can alternatively be done simply using facial landmarks. The cuspid bisector closely corresponds to an imaginary line drawn from the tip of the cuspid to the pupil of the eye on the opposite side of the body. Using this technique, all that remains is ensuring that the entire receptor is fully exposed by the PID.

region with minimal distortion of the teeth and include the interproximal region of the first bicuspid and distal of the cuspid. If an instrument is not used to hold the receptor in place, one of the patient's fingers may be used to press the receptor up against the lingual side of the bicuspids. Generally, having the patient use the hand opposite to the side being exposed reduces the likelihood of that hand blocking the x-ray beam. If the operator uses a PSP plate, a gentle finger pressure should be used to reduce bending of the receptor that would cause distortion of the image. The horizontal angulation of the x-ray beam should be aimed through the contact area between the bicuspids and cuspid to minimize overlapping of these teeth. To determine the correct positive vertical angulation of the PID, the operator must visualize the plane of the receptor and the long axis of the bicuspids and then bisect these two lines. The central ray of the PID should then be aimed perpendicular to this imaginary bisecting line with the lower edge of the PID extending beyond the edge of the receptor. Once again approximation of the correct vertical angle can alternatively be done with facial landmarks. The bicuspid bisector closely corresponds to an imaginary line drawn from the buccal cusp of the bicuspid to the midpoint between the patient's eyes directly superficial to the skeletal landmark referred to as *nasion* ☢. Using this technique, all that remains for the operator is to ensure that the entire receptor is fully exposed by the PID.

Maxillary bicuspid bisecting angle projection

Area of interest: First and second bicuspids.

Receptor size: No. 2.

Position: The receptor must be rotated so that the long dimension of the receptor is orientated *horizontally*. The operator should position the receptor towards the midline of the palate, which is the deepest area of the palatal vault, and bring the anterior edge of the receptor up to the distal of the cuspid. This will assist capturing the apical

Maxillary molar bisecting angle projection

Area of interest: First, second and third molars.

Receptor size: No. 2.

Position: Similar to the bicuspid view, the receptor must be rotated so that the long dimension of the receptor is orientated *horizontally* in the patient's mouth. The operator should position the top of the receptor towards the midline of the palate and bring the anterior edge of the receptor up to the distal of the second bicuspid. The receptor may not be long enough to capture the entire molar region desired in a single view. If a full mouth series of images is being performed, the operator may determine that the bicuspid view has already captured the first molar. Consequently, the operator can then position the receptor further posteriorly to capture the tuberosity region along with the second and third molars. To capture the tuberosity region, it is recommended that the operator position the receptor initially in the bicuspid area and then request the patient to move the receptor with their own hand as far posteriorly as they can tolerate. This will avoid unnecessary retakes as the operator will know that the patient has already placed the receptor as far posteriorly as possible. If the tuberosity region is still not visible, the operator should resort to exposing an extraoral image, such as a panoramic image, if available. If an instrument is not used to hold the receptor in place, the patient's finger may be used to press the receptor up against the lingual side of the molars. If the operator uses a PSP plate, a gentle finger pressure should be used to reduce bending of the receptor that would cause distortion of the image. Generally, having the patient use the hand opposite to the side being exposed reduces the likelihood of that hand blocking the x-ray beam. The horizontal angulation of the x-ray beam should be aimed through the contact area between the molars to minimize overlapping of these teeth. To determine the correct positive vertical angulation of the PID, the operator must visualize the plane of the receptor and the long axis of the multirooted molars and then bisect these two lines. The central ray of the PID should then be aimed perpendicular to this imaginary bisecting line with the lower edge of the PID extending beyond the edge of the receptor. The vertical angle of the maxillary molars tends to be slightly greater than the premolars angulation. The following suggestion should not to be used as an absolute angle but preselecting a 30–40° positive vertical angle of the PID in relation to the occlusal plane often works.

Mandibular incisor bisecting angle projection

Area of interest: Incisors.

Receptor size: No. 1 (preferable for ease of placement) or no. 2.

Position: The long dimension of the receptor should be positioned *vertically* and parallel to the labial surfaces of the incisors. Note that in the anterior region of the mouth, the receptor can be placed on the dorsal surface of the tongue. This often will allow the operator to fully seat the receptor in the patient's mouth and still capture the apical region. Furthermore, placing the receptor further posteriorly away from the lingual surfaces of the teeth also reduces receptor discomfort and typically allows the patient to fully bite together. The horizontal angulation of the x-ray beam should be aimed through the contact area between the incisors to minimize overlapping of these teeth. The operator must then determine the correct negative vertical angulation of the PID by first visualizing the plane of the receptor and the long axes of the incisors. The angle that these two lines form must be visually bisected. The central ray of the PID should then be aimed perpendicular to this imaginary line with the lower edge of the PID extending beyond the edge of the receptor. Because the mandibular incisors are typically quite narrow, the operator may be able to capture all four incisors in one image. However, if a portion of the left or right lateral incisor is cut off this view, the operator should next image the cuspid. The lateral incisor often is visible on the cuspid view. In so doing, it will eliminate the need for an additional lateral incisor exposure.

Mandibular cuspid bisecting angle projection

Area of interest: Cuspid and lateral incisor.

Receptor size: No. 2.

Position: The long dimension of the receptor should be positioned *vertically* and parallel to the labial surface of the cuspid. Placing the receptor further away from the lingual surfaces of the teeth will reduce discomfort. The horizontal angulation of the x-ray beam should be aimed toward the contact area between the cuspid and first bicuspid to minimize overlapping of these two teeth. Constriction and curvature of the mandibular arch will undoubtedly result in some superimposition of the first bicuspid onto the distal surface of the cuspid. However, the distal contact of the cuspid should be visible either on the bicuspid bitewing or periapical images. The correct negative vertical angulation of the PID can be determined by first visualizing the plane of the receptor and the long axis of the cuspid. The angle that these two lines form must be visually bisected. The central ray of the PID should then be aimed perpendicular to this imaginary line with the lower edge of the PID extending beyond the edge of the receptor.

Note: The mucosa in this area of the oral cavity tends to be particularly sensitive and the patient may not tolerate fully seating the receptor.

Mandibular bicuspid bisecting angle projection

Area of interest: First and second bicuspids.
   Receptor size: No. 2.
   Position: For this projection, the long dimension of the receptor must be positioned *horizontally*. Intraorally, the receptor should be aligned parallel to both the buccal surfaces and the long axes of the teeth. Because the long dimension of the receptor is positioned horizontally to capture the posterior teeth, it cannot be placed onto the dorsal surface of the tongue. In this scenario, the tongue would prevent the shorter height of the receptor to be seated far enough inferiorly to capture the entire apical region. Consequently, the instrument must be positioned between the patient's tongue and next to the alveolar ridge, which may be quite uncomfortable for the

patient and often will result in missing the mesial portion of the first bicuspid. Using a PSP plate permits gentle bending of the receptor away from the sensitive mucosa, thus allowing it to be placed more anteriorly to hopefully capture the mesial of the first bicuspid. Care must be taken not to overbend a PSP plate as it may become permanently bent and likely compromise future imaging. The horizontal angulation of the x-ray beam should be aimed toward the contact area between the first and second bicuspids to minimize overlapping of these two teeth. The correct negative vertical angulation of the PID can be determined by first visualizing the plane of the receptor and the long axes of the bicuspids. The angle that these two lines form must be visually bisected. The central ray of the PID should then be aimed perpendicular to this imaginary line with the lower edge of the PID extending beyond the edge of the receptor. The long axes of the bicuspids are normally almost vertical, thus very little angulation of the PID will be required, possibly up to 15° of negative vertical angulation. However, the length of the bicuspids often matches or exceeds the length of the receptor when positioned horizontally. Consequently, the operator may need to compromise and intentionally overangulate the PID vertically to project the image of the apical region onto the receptor. This will distort the image and likely cut off a portion of the crown(s), but will at least capture the periapical region. The missing coronal region(s) should be visible on a bicuspid bitewing image.

Mandibular molar bisecting angle projection

Area of interest: First, second and third molars.
   Receptor size: No. 2.
   Position: Similar to the bicuspid view, the receptor must be rotated so the long dimension of the receptor is orientated *horizontally* and should be positioned between the patient's tongue and the alveolar ridge. It may not be quite

as uncomfortable for a patient as the bicuspid view as the receptor is positioned further from the very sensitive anterior mucosa. The anterior aspect of the receptor should be positioned at the middle of the second bicuspid tooth to ensure visualization of the mesial contact area of the first molar. Similar to the maxillary molar view, the receptor may not be long enough to capture the retromolar region. In a full mouth series of images, the bicuspid view typically captures the first molar. Consequently, the operator can position the receptor further posteriorly to capture the retromolar region. Once again, to avoid unnecessary retakes, the operator should position the receptor initially in the bicuspid region and then request the patient to move the receptor as far back as they can tolerate with their own hand. After doing so, if the retromolar region is still not captured on the image, the operator should expose an extraoral image, such as a panoramic image, if available. The horizontal angulation of the x-ray beam should be aimed toward the contact area between the first and second molars to minimize overlapping of these two teeth. The correct negative vertical angulation of the PID can be determined by first visualizing the plane of the receptor and the long axes of the molars. The angle that these two lines form must be visually bisected. The central ray of the PID should then be aimed perpendicular to this imaginary line with the lower edge of the PID extending beyond the edge of the receptor. The long axes of the molars, like the bicuspids, are typically almost vertical, thus very little angulation of the PID will be required, possibly 10–15° of negative vertical angulation. Similar to the bicuspids, the length of the molars often will match or exceed the length of the receptor when positioned horizontally. Consequently, the operator may need to compromise and intentionally overangulate the PID vertically to project the image of the periapical regions onto the receptor. This will distort the image and likely cut off a portion of the crown(s), but will at least capture the periapical regions. The missing coronal region(s) should be visible on a molar bitewing image.

3. BITEWING TECHNIQUE

The objectives of a bitewing projection are ideally to visualize open interproximal contacts and the crest of the alveolar bone of both arches. A conventional full mouth series of x-ray images often includes a set of four bitewings. Bitewing instruments are available. Many operators prefer to only use a disposable tab for the patient to bite down upon to hold the receptor in place, without having any additional alignment device (i.e. ring) attached. An experienced operator may use a freehand technique that allows the operator more flexibility in orientating the PID both horizontally and vertically. An operator with little experience initially should use a bitewing instrument with an alignment device attached. Regardless of the technique used, it is recommended that the operator align the patient's occlusal plane parallel to the floor, particularly if the operator is performing it freehand. This will allow easier determination of the correct horizontal and vertical position of the PID. To avoid overlapping the coronal contacts, the horizontal angulation must be aimed between the contact points of the adjacent teeth (Fig. K13). Tooth rotation or crowding will complicate visualizing multiple open contacts on a single bitewing image. Consequently, the operator may be required to take multiple

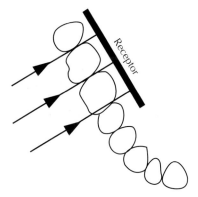

Fig. K13 Illustration of the proper horizontal angulation to separate (i.e. open) adjacent surface contacts.

bitewings, each one using a slightly different horizontal angulation to eliminate overlapping of specific contacts. Overlapped contacts can obscure caries, fractures, etc. Why are periapical images not adequate for viewing bone levels? The vertical angulation typically used, regardless of whether paralleling or bisecting angle techniques were used, are greater. Vertical angulation for bitewings is minimal (i.e. 0–8° positive vertical). Consequently, the relationship of bone level to tooth position is maintained on a bitewing image. An exception can be the mandibular molar periapical image which may require almost no vertical angulation of the x-ray beam.

Bicuspid bitewing (Fig. K14)

Areas of interest: A bicuspid bitewing positioned to include the distal of the cuspid anteriorly.

Receptor size: No. 2 for adult dentition, nos. 1 or 0 for children.

Position: For this projection, the long dimension of the receptor must be attached *horizontally* and should be aligned parallel to the buccal surfaces of the teeth. Similar to the periapical technique, the receptor must be positioned between the patient's tongue and next to the alveolar ridge. Using a PSP plate

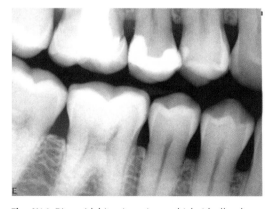

Fig. K14 Bicuspid bitewing view, which ideally shows both the maxillary and mandibular bicuspids with open contacts and the height of the alveolar crestal bone.

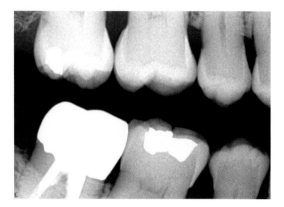

Fig. K15 Molar bitewing view.

permits bending of the plate allowing it to be placed more anteriorly to capture the mesial of the cuspid.

Molar bitewing (Fig. K15)

Position: Similar to the bicuspid projection, the long dimension of the receptor must be positioned *horizontally* and should be aligned parallel to the buccal surfaces of the teeth and positioned between the patient's tongue and the alveolar ridge. It may not be quite as uncomfortable for a patient as the bicuspid view as the receptor is positioned further from the very sensitive anterior mucosa. The anterior aspect of the receptor should be positioned to include the distal of the second bicuspid tooth to ensure visualization of the mesial contact area of the first molar. Unlike a periapical view, the posterior extent of the receptor does not need to extend all the way to the retromolar region because bitewings focus on interproximal contacts of adjacent teeth.

Anterior bitewing projection (Fig. K16)

Position: Bitewings in the anterior region are difficult to perform, particularly with solid-state receptors as a result of the receptor's bulk and rigidity. However, using a thinner, flexible

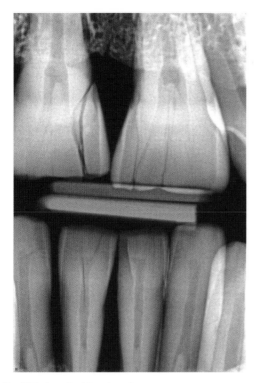

Fig. K16 Anterior bitewing view.

PSP plate allows the operator to more easily position the receptor in the anterior region to acquire a bitewing of the incisors. Generally, the same principles that were used for aligning the bicuspid and molar regions also apply here. However in the anterior region, the coronal portions of the maxillary and mandibular incisors are in different planes. Consequently, the receptor cannot be aligned perfectly parallel to the crowns of both the maxillary and mandibular incisors simultaneously. This will result in some distortion of the bitewing image. Imaging the maxillary and mandibular teeth independently can eliminate this problem.

4. DISTAL OBLIQUE TECHNIQUE

The distal oblique technique is primarily a standard molar projection using the bisecting angle technique but with a definite modification to the horizontal angulation of the PID and the receptor position (Fig. K17). This technique may compromise the overall quality of the image but it can provide additional information that may otherwise be unattainable. For example, if the operator encounters a patient with a hypersensitive gag reflex, it may be impossible to position the receptor far enough posteriorly to image the entire tooth or region of interest.

For the maxillary third molar region, the operator should begin by positioning the receptor in the typical premolar region where the patient is less likely to gag. If the instrument has a ring for aligning the PID, the operator should remove it prior to insertion into the patient's mouth as it may interfere with the modified PID position. Upon insertion, the operator should gently turn the distal end of the receptor away from the teeth of interest so that it is now angled across the midline toward the opposite side, while the anterior end of the receptor is left unchanged. There is not a universal horizontal angulation to use. Aiming the PID from the distal direction toward the receptor at approximately a 45° horizontal angle should be adequate. Unfortunately it may require a trial and error approach. This will project the image of the teeth and the maxillary tuberosity region anteriorly onto the receptor. It will also likely result in the coronal portions of the teeth being overlapped. Overlapped crowns should not be a major concern if there is a molar bitewing image to view. In this projection, the roots and apices that were not captured using standard procedures should now be visible.

The distal oblique technique for the mandibular third molar region is slightly different to that of the maxillary molar projection. If the instrument has a ring for the aligning the PID, the operator should remove it prior to insertion into the patient's mouth. For the mandible, because of physical constraints of the tongue, the receptor must be positioned between the tongue and the alveolar ridge and aligned parallel to the latter, as in the

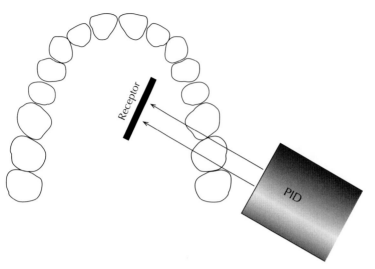

Fig. K17 Diagram demonstrating the distal oblique technique. PID, position indicating device.

paralleling and bisecting angle techniques. The operator must then slide the receptor as far posteriorly as the patient will permit. Similar to the maxillary molar distal oblique method, the horizontal angulation of the PID will be aimed obliquely and from the distal end of the region of interest. Aiming the PID at approximately a 45° horizontal angle toward the receptor should work. The oblique angulation will project the image more anteriorly onto the receptor. Similar to the maxillary projection, the coronal portions of adjacent teeth will likely be overlapped, but the individual roots and their apices should be visible on the image.

5. OCCLUSAL IMAGING TECHNIQUE

The term *occlusal technique* refers to the physical position of the intraoral receptor only. The intraoral receptor is aligned horizontally between the occlusal surfaces of the maxillary and mandibular teeth. For this reason, it is also called the "sandwich technique" because it mimics placing a sandwich in one's mouth. This technique can be performed with any size receptor. When film was the standard receptor,

an occlusal-size film was marketed; its physical size resembled a playing card. Today, PSP plates can be purchased comparable in size to an occlusal film for a reasonable price. Unfortunately, the limited need for *occlusal images* ☢ in private practice makes it impractical for manufacturers to produce a comparably sized solid-state receptor from a cost perspective. However, a no. 2 solid-state receptor can still be used to expose an occlusal image. The size of the receptor does not differentiate the principles of the occlusal technique, it merely controls the amount of real estate visible on an image. When utilizing the occlusal technique, a larger receptor is preferable as it will obviously image a larger area compared with a smaller receptor.

An occlusal image gives the practitioner a bucco-lingual perspective of the region that is not visible on a standard periapical or panoramic view. This is particularly beneficial in localizing impactions and sialoliths. In addition, an occlusal projection may permit imaging when periapical or bitewing images are impossible to acquire, such as in a case of *trismus* ☢. If the patient is not able to open wide enough to allow positioning a receptor attached to an instrument, then the operator can request the patient to use their own hand to slide the receptor in place. Since this technique requires minimal mouth opening, it avoids the operator unnecessarily traumatizing the patient further. Occlusal images will offer additional diagnostic information, especially if extraoral imaging equipment is unavailable. It is recommended that the operator select a posterior periapical setting initially and then adjust the exposure settings either up or down if a retake is necessary.

Maxillary occlusal projection

The maxillary occlusal image requires the same bisecting angle technique that is used for periapical images (Figs K18 and K19). Regardless of the size of the receptor selected for this procedure, the operator must slide the receptor over the area of interest. If this is the posterior right region, the receptor should be slid as far posteriorly as possible and offset to the right side. If the area of interest is the anterior region, then the receptor should be aligned more anteriorly. In this situation, if a no. 2 receptor is used, it may be preferable to position the long dimension of the receptor sideways from right to left. The operator must decide which orientation of the receptor is best for each particular situation. Using the bisecting angle principles, the PID should be aimed at a right angle to the bisector of the angle formed by the receptor and the long axes of the teeth. Generally, the vertical angle of the PID will be approximately 65° positive from the occlusal plane. For edentulous patients the operator may use the buccal or lingual plates of the edentulous ridge in lieu of roots to determine a bisector. Attempting to align the PID at a right angle to the receptor is usually not recommended because of superimposition of the cranium over the area of interest and the need for a much higher exposure to penetrate the additional skeletal structures to acquire a diagnostic image.

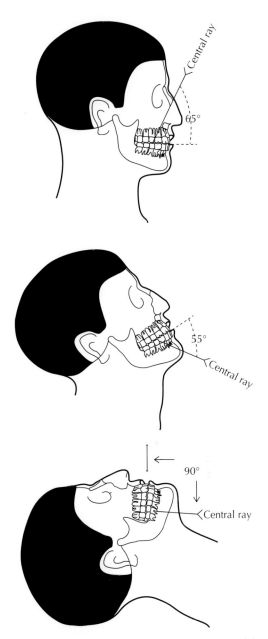

Fig. K18 Illustrations demonstrating the principles of the occlusal technique

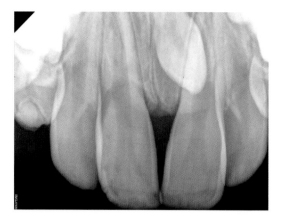

Fig. K19 Occlusal view of the maxillary anterior teeth.

Mandibular occlusal projection

Unlike the maxilla, where superimposition of the cranium interferes with performing a right angle projection, the anatomy of the mandibular region permits using either a bisecting angle or a right angle projection (Figs K18 and K20). A right angle projection is easily accomplished by placing the receptor in the region of interest and then directing the PID at 90° to the receptor from beneath the mandible. This perpendicular angulation is more easily attained when the patient tips their head backwards, thereby allowing the tubehead to lie lower down along the patient's chest.

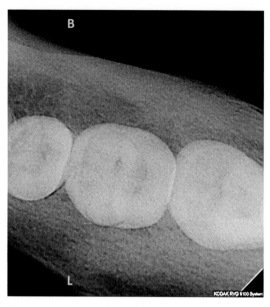

Fig. K20 Occlusal view of the mandibular molar region (B, buccal aspect; L, lingual aspect).

A bisecting angle view also requires placement of the receptor in the region of interest and the PID aimed at a right angle to the bisector of the angle formed by the receptor and the long axes of the teeth. Generally, the vertical angle of the PID will be approximately 55° negative from the occlusal plane. For edentulous patients the operator may use the buccal or lingual plates of the edentulous ridge in lieu of roots to determine the bisector.

L Intraoral Technique Errors

Regardless of whether the paralleling or bisecting angle technique is used, several factors must be incorporated to acquire good diagnostic images. This includes: (i) patient and receptor positioning; (ii) proper vertical and horizontal angulation of the PID; and (iii) correct selection of the exposure settings (i.e. mA, kVp and exposure time).

The following technical errors are discussed in this section:

1. Cone-cut
2. Apex missing
3. Elongation
4. Foreshortening
5. Overlapped contacts
6. Missing contact
7. Overexposure and underexposure
8. Motion artifact
9. Foreign object

Cone-cut

A *cone-cut* refers to an unexposed area of varying size on the periphery of an intraoral image (Fig. L1). For whatever reason, it is a result of the x-ray beam not being properly aligned with the receptor. The part of the receptor extending outside the beam of radiation will not be exposed. Historically, the PID has been called a "cone." The unexposed area appears blank as if it was "cut," hence the combined term "cone-cut." Even though PID has generally replaced the term cone, the term cone-cut has remained and it has not been updated to a "PID-cut." To confirm that the blank area is a cone-cut, the outline of the blank area must either be a curved line from using a round PID or a straight line resulting from using a rectangular PID.

There are different causes for cone-cut images. Many teaching institutions commonly use intraoral RINN XCP™ for intraoral imaging. This instrument kit may include three different set-ups; each set-up is used for a specific purpose (i.e. anterior periapical, posterior periapical and bitewing projections). If the operator uses the wrong aiming ring or assembles the instruments incorrectly, it will result in a cone-cut. When using a rectangular PID, it must be very accurately aligned with the surface of the receptor as the rectangular beam size closely matches the receptor size. Occasionally the PID may drift away from the instrument after the operator properly aligns it with the receptor. Over time the weight of the tubehead can loosen the bracket arm, allowing it to drift

Fundamentals of Oral and Maxillofacial Radiology, First Edition. J. Sean Hubar.
© 2017 John Wiley & Sons, Inc. Published 2017 by John Wiley & Sons, Inc.
Companion website: www.wiley.com/go/hubar/radiology

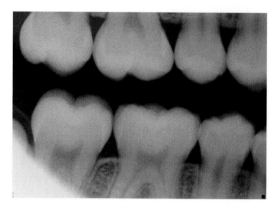

Fig. L1 Cone-cut (highlighted).

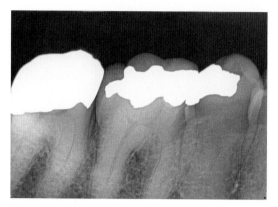

Fig. L2 Missing apices can be due to the receptor not being positioned properly, vertical underangulation or long root length.

slightly. In this scenario, the operator may align the PID correctly and walk out of the operatory without observing the drift of the PID. The patient is exposed and the result is a cone-cut image.

Note: If the operator attempts the occlusal technique using a large PSP plate, an unexposed area will frequently appear on the image. This should not be considered an operator error as it is directly the result of the receptor size being larger than the x-ray beam size.

Apex missing

If an apex of a tooth is absent from an image, the receptor is not positioned far enough apically to image the entire tooth (Fig. L2). Using the paralleling technique, the operator can reposition the receptor further away from the lingual surfaces of the teeth. In the mandible, the patient's tongue may force the receptor up against the alveolar ridge. Pressing the receptor up against the tongue may permit the operator to push the receptor away from the ridge and thereby permit the receptor to be seated more apically. In the maxilla, the midline of the palatal vault is typically the deepest aspect and allows a greater opportunity to capture the

apex on the image. However, a shallow palate and a palatal torus are definite contraindications for the paralleling technique. Either obstacle can prevent the receptor from being positioned far enough apically to capture an apex, leaving the operator with no option but to intentionally foreshorten the image with vertical overangulation. The bisecting angle technique can be used more effectively in this scenario. The operator should slide the receptor along the palate, leaving a minimum of receptor surface extending beyond the occlusal edge. Still failing to capture the apex will require the operator to use extraoral imaging techniques, such as a panoramic view to visualize the apical region.

An unavoidable cause of a missing apex occurs when a tooth is clinically longer than the length of the receptor. In the anterior region, substituting a no. 1 receptor with a no. 2 receptor will provide additional height for acquiring the apices. The maxillary cuspid generally is the longest tooth in the arch and, as a result, it often poses logistical problems in attempts to image it entirely. To accommodate the anatomy in the posterior regions of the maxilla and mandible, the long dimension of a no. 2 receptor must be positioned horizontally. Substituting a no. 2 receptor with a smaller no. 1 receptor and orientating it vertically generally will not work. Failure to capture the apical region may require the operator to intentionally vertically overangulate the PID or to resort to extraoral imaging techniques.

Elongation

Underangulation of the PID will elongate the length of the tooth, which may project the apex of the tooth off the receptor (Fig. L3). To correct this, the operator must now increase the *vertical angulation* ☢ of the PID, taking care not to overcompensate and overangulate the PID. *Elongation* is a common bisecting angle technique error. Even for an experienced operator performing the bisecting angle technique often is a trial and error effort. If the operator is using a PSP plate, care must be taken not to use too much pressure to hold it in position intraorally.

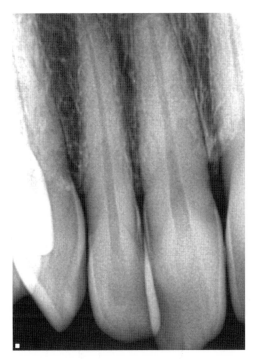

Fig. L3 Elongation of the image as a result of inadequate vertical angulation.

This type of receptor is very flexible and pressure can cause it to bend, which will elongate the image. Elongation caused by underangulation of the PID while using a paralleling instrument is physically difficult to do.

Foreshortening

Foreshortening will make a tooth appear shorter than it should be (Fig. L4). When is foreshortening problematic? Accurate measurement of tooth length is critical for performing, for example, endodontic procedures. Excessive vertical angulation of the PID with either the paralleling or bisecting angle technique will foreshorten the image (see Fig. V1). If the receptor is positioned intraorally and the operator observes that the PID is in a steep vertical position, the PID likely needs to be repositioned. If it is not recognized and subsequently a retake is required, the operator should reposition the receptor further away from the teeth. This positioning adjustment will reduce the vertical angulation and result in a more accurate representation of the teeth. The operator must also understand that a steep vertical angulation will result in a greater *attenuation* ☢ of the x-ray beam because the x rays are traveling through more

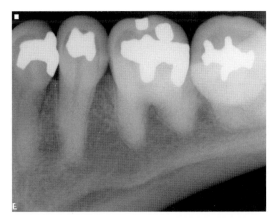

Fig. L4 Foreshortening of the image as a result of excessive vertical angulation.

tissue. Consequently, a foreshortened image may also appear somewhat underexposed. Correcting the vertical angulation alone may be all that is required to increase the density of the new image. The point being, the operator must not automatically increase the exposure settings without first taking attenuation into consideration.

Overlapped contacts

Incorrect *horizontal angulation* ♣♠ of the PID causes overlapping of the interproximal surfaces of adjacent teeth (Fig. L5). It should be noted that it may occur either from overangling the PID either from the mesial or from the distal direction toward the region being imaged. The objective is to aim the x-ray beam directly between the teeth. Factors such as tooth rotation and tooth crowding may make it impossible to achieve or at the very least it would require multiple images to accommodate all of these irregularities. Immediately after the exposure is processed, the operator should examine the x-ray image to determine what horizontal angulation was used. The key is to check for both the open and the overlapped contacts. Why is it that some of the proximal contacts are open while others are overlapped? Each open

contact indicates that the x-ray beam passed between those two teeth. However, the shape and orientation of those teeth showing overlapped contacts must be different and therefore require a different horizontal angulation to open them. For example, if a bicuspid bitewing image shows separation only between the cuspid and first bicuspid, and all of the other teeth distal to them are overlapped, the PID needs to be aimed more from the distal direction. In essence this means that the PID must be horizontally swung around more to the side of the patient. Doing so should open up the contacts between the two bicuspids, but will likely now overlap the previously open contact between the cuspid and first bicuspid area. Beware that overcompensation of the horizontal angulation from the distal direction will also produce undesired overlapping. Separation of contacts is critical for the diagnosis of interproximal caries and the assessment of mesial and distal margins of restorations on bitewing images.

Missing contacts

In general, if the receptor position is too far anterior or too far posterior intraorally it can easily cut off proximal contacts surfaces (Fig. L6).

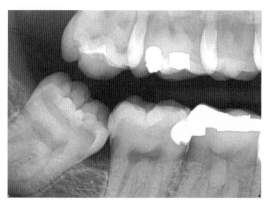

Fig. L5 Overlapped contacts caused by incorrect horizontal angulation (see Fig. K13).

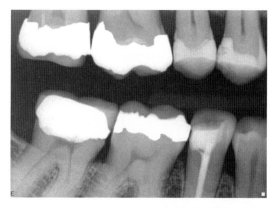

Fig. L6 Absent surface: missing mesial surface of the mandibular first bicuspid as a result of the receptor not being positioned far enough anteriorly. Note that proper horizontal angulation produced open contacts.

A very common problematic area is the mandibular cuspid and first bicuspid region. The anterior curvature of the dental arch can make this area almost impossible to properly image, especially when using bulky solid-state receptors. Compounding this problem, all solid-state sensors contain a *dead space* ☢ of up to a few millimeters inside the anterior edge of the receptor. The outer casing of the receptor may appear to be far enough anterior but the solid-state circuits contained within it will not capture the extreme anterior edge. Dead space is not a concern on PSP plates.

Overexposure and underexposure

In general, excessive x-ray production will result in an *overexposed* ☢ image and, conversely, inadequate x-ray production will produce an *underexposed* ☢ image (Fig. L7). It is important to understand that standardized exposure settings are not universal for multiple reasons. Factors to consider in determining the proper exposure settings are the physical size of the patient, whether you are imaging the anterior region versus the posterior region or the maxillary teeth versus the mandibular teeth, the type of receptor being used, and the distance and angulation of the PID toward the receptor. Some intraoral x-ray units only allow the operator to modify the exposure time. Consequently, increasing or decreasing the exposure time may be the operator's only option. Finally, one should also be aware that the total radiation output from the x-ray tube will gradually diminish with usage.

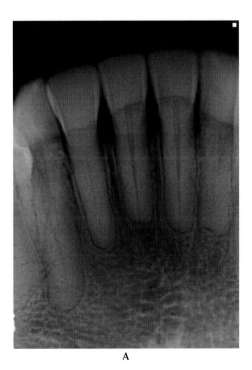

A

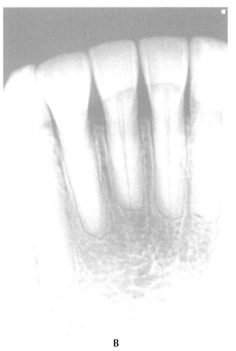

B

Fig. L7 A. Dark image: overexposure as a result of excessive radiation exposure. B. Light image: underexposure.

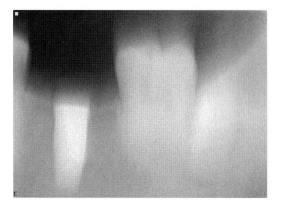

Fig. L8 Blurred image due to patient movement.

Motion artifact

Ideally, the patient, tubehead and receptor all remain motionless during the exposure. Movement of any of these in any combination will reduce the sharpness of the image (Fig. L8). There is a difference between movements of the receptor alone versus movement of the patient's head. For example, the patient may use the tongue to reposition the receptor during the exposure and yet keep their head steady. At other times, the patient and receptor will move in tandem if the patient turns their head. Movement of the receptor or the patient's head during the exposure will likely produce noticeable blurriness of the image, while motion effects produced by a drifting x-ray tubehead alone will be more subtle. The tubehead would have to move significantly during the exposure to cause noticeable image unsharpness. However a more significant consequence could be a cone-cut image.

Foreign object

Patients should be instructed to remove dentures and eyeglasses prior to intraoral imaging. Unlike extraoral imaging, jewelry worn

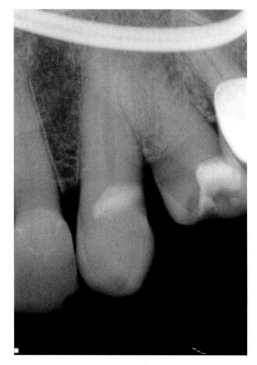

Fig. L9 Eyeglass frame (highlighted).

around the neck or in the ears may remain in place for intraoral imaging as they will be outside the field of view. However, the metal framework of partial dentures and eyeglass frames may be projected over the apices of the teeth, which may necessitate retaking the image (Fig. L9). Plastic protective eyewear typically does not pose a problem and may be left on the patient during intraoral imaging. Overangulation of the PID may project the metal arm of the intraoral receptor holder over the incisal edges of teeth (Fig. L10). Fingers should also be kept out of view (Fig. L11).

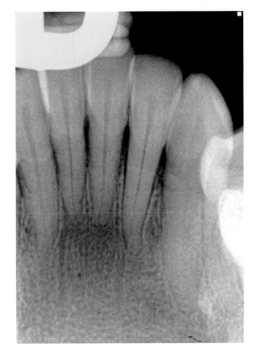

Fig. L10 Receptor holder (highlighted).

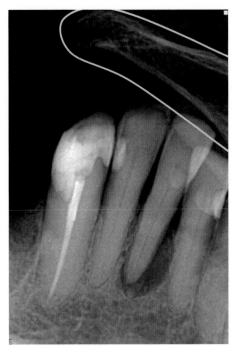

Fig. L11 Fingertip (highlighted).

M

Extraoral Imaging Techniques

Extraoral images are acquired when the image receptor is positioned outside of the patient's mouth. Extraoral images are particularly beneficial for patients requiring orthodontic treatment, dental implants and oral surgical procedures. Typical extraoral x-ray images include panoramic, cephalometric and CBCT projections.

1. PANORAMIC IMAGING

According to the Oxford English dictionary a "panorama" is defined as an unbroken view of the whole region surrounding an observer. In dentistry, a panoramic x-ray image is a single, unobstructed image of the entire mandible and maxilla (Fig. M1). At the outset, the author wishes to acknowledge that a discussion of the physics of the complicated imaging equipment involved is beyond the scope of this book.

Panoramic x-ray units have become ubiquitous in dental offices. The first commercially available panoramic unit was introduced in the 1950s. The latest evolution of panoramic x-ray units has substituted a digital image receptor in lieu of a film receptor. Basic physical differences amongst panoramic units include whether the patient is seated or standing during the procedure, bite-block design, exposure controls, availability of a cephalometric attachment, etc. Today, more sophisticated panoramic units also have limited cone-beam technology capability directly built into them.

The primary component of any panoramic x-ray unit is a horizontal rotating arm that houses at one end the x-ray tube, and at the other end an image receptor. The generated x rays are immediately collimated into a narrow, vertical beam. The x-ray beam is usually only a few millimeters wide and has enough vertical height to expose both the mandibular and maxillary arches. During the exposure, the horizontal assembly rotates completely around the patient's head. Of significance is the fact that the patient is only exposed to a narrow beam of radiation at any one moment. This explains why a patient typically receives less radiation from a larger *panoramic image* ☢ compared with a full mouth series of intraoral images. Also, unlike intraoral images where an entire image will be blurred by patient motion during the exposure, only a limited area of a panoramic image will be blurred if there is a momentary period of patient movement. Patient motion only affects the area of the panoramic image

Fundamentals of Oral and Maxillofacial Radiology, First Edition. J. Sean Hubar.
© 2017 John Wiley & Sons, Inc. Published 2017 by John Wiley & Sons, Inc.
Companion website: www.wiley.com/go/hubar/radiology

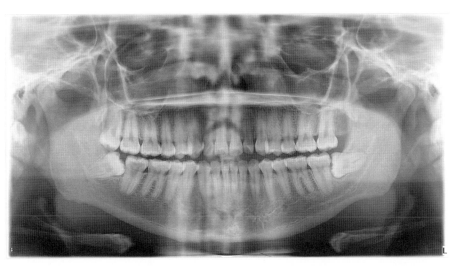

Fig. M1 Panoramic image.

exposed during that period of time. Once the patient becomes still again, the remaining area of the image will not be affected.

Positioning the patient

Accurate patient positioning is critical to acquire a diagnostic panoramic image (Fig. M2). Most modern panoramic units are designed with the patient in a standing position for the x-ray exposure. The patient must be guided by the operator into the gantry of the unit. Generally, there will be a bite-block of some fashion that the operator should instruct the patient to bite onto using their maxillary and mandibular incisors. An alternative chin rest often is provided by the manufacturer for properly positioning fully edentulous patients.

Head positioning utilizes three anatomic planes – the sagittal, transverse and coronal planes – and controls the side to side, anterior–posterior and inferior–superior positions of the mandible and maxilla. The patient's jaws are guided into a *focal trough* ☢. A focal trough is

also called the "zone of sharpness." Positioning the patient within the focal trough will result in optimum diagnostic quality of the image; failure to do so will result in varying degrees of image distortion. The focal trough is generally horseshoe-shaped (i.e. U shape), with the open end located in the posterior region. For every model of panoramic unit, the focal trough may vary in size and shape. Panoramic units typically use laser lines that are projected onto the facial soft tissues to assist the operator in positioning the patient's head. Be cognizant that the actual outline of the focal trough is invisible to the operator as it is not marked on the exterior of the x-ray unit.

The Frankfort horizontal plane is used to determine the proper inferior-superior position of the patient's head. It is formed by an imaginary line that extends between the external auditory meatus and the inferior margin (floor) of the orbit. This plane is often considered the normal carrying position for the head when a person is facing forward and standing upright. If a patient's chin is tipped too far down in the panoramic unit, it will collapse the image size of the dental arch, while tipping the chin too far

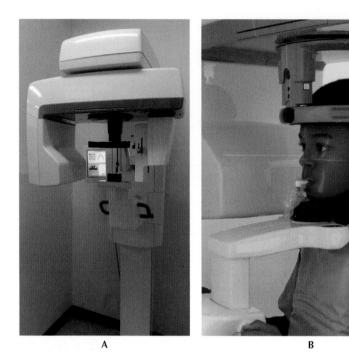

A   B

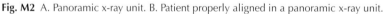

Fig. M2 A. Panoramic x-ray unit. B. Patient properly aligned in a panoramic x-ray unit.

upwards may result in the posterior aspect of the ramus and condyle being cut off the image.

The mid-sagittal plane is used to center the patient's head laterally in the x-ray unit. It is intended to eliminate the head being off-center or turned to one side. The operator typically relies on soft tissue landmarks using the midline of the nose and the midpoint between the eyes for positioning the patient. However, the soft tissue midline and the skeletal midline may not coincide with one another. In this scenario, using the soft tissue midline would result in distortion of the image. Whenever a patient's skeletal midline is positioned off-center, there will be magnification on one side of the dentition and the opposite side will be simultaneously demagnified. Prior to the exposure, the operator should also confirm the mid-sagittal positioning by viewing the patient's head from the back as the mid-sagittal line may be centered correctly on their face but the posterior

aspect of their head may be off-center and may need to be repositioned by the operator.

The mandibular cuspid is typically used as the guide to properly position the patient antero-posteriorly in a panoramic unit. A patient positioned too far anteriorly will result in demagnification of the anterior teeth on the image. Conversely, if the patient is positioned too far posteriorly, it will magnify the image size of the anterior dentition. Positioning completely edentulous patients is slightly more challenging although the same protocol applies. Manufacturers typically have modified bite-blocks or chin cups for positioning edentulous patients. However, if a modified bite-block is not available, the operator can still use a standard bite-block. In this situation, the operator should ask the patient to gently close their lips around the tip of the bite-block. Use of the Frankfort horizontal position and the mid-sagittal plane is the same. However, for antero-posterior positioning, the operator can use the corner of the lips as a virtual cuspid. For all patients, partial dentures should be removed prior to placing the patient in the panoramic unit.

Exposure settings

All panoramic units allow the operator to adjust the milliamperage and kilovoltage settings. Unlike intraoral x-ray units, the panoramic exposure time is always fixed and averages approximately 20 s. Panoramic exposure time is in fact the time it takes for the tubehead and receptor to rotate around the patient's head and may vary slightly from one manufacturer's x-ray unit to another. Whether the operator manually selects exposure settings or permits the x-ray unit to automatically determine the exposure, familiarity with the functioning of the panoramic unit will ultimately remove a lot of the guesswork and produce the best images.

Advantages and disadvantages

Advantages

1. Image content
2. Image context
3. Patient comfort
4. Efficiency
5. Bitewing mode
6. Dose reduction
7. Cost effectiveness
8. Standing position versus seated style panoramic unit

Image content

A single panoramic image includes the entire oral region, often including additional structures outside the field of view of conventional intraoral images. These may include the temporomandibular joint, maxillary sinuses, nasal cavity, hyoid bone, etc.

Image context

A famous phrase of psychologist Kurt Koffka, "The whole is *other* than the sum of the parts" is often incorrectly translated as "The whole is *greater* than the sum of its parts." One can relate this to x-ray images by defining a panoramic image as the "whole" and intraoral images as the "parts." A panoramic image relates the physical relationships of anatomic structures to one another much better than a disjointed full mouth series of intraoral images. In essence a panoramic image is a *gestalt* ☢ of the oral region.

Patient comfort

Unless a patient is extremely claustrophobic, a panoramic projection is a very comfortable procedure to have performed. Patients generally are required to stand upright, rest their chin on a platform and bite onto the tip of a plastic rod. This may also be the only viable option for imaging the dentition of a patient with a hypersensitive gag reflex.

Efficiency

In comparison to the cumulative time it takes to expose a full mouth series of intraoral images, the time to acquire a panoramic image is very brief, at approximately 20 s. For the majority of patients a 20 s exposure time is inconsequential. However, the exposure time can be problematic for patients suffering from any type of tremor who may be unable to hold steady for that long. In this case, intraoral images may actually be preferable where the exposures can be intermittent, very brief and ideally timed to counter patient movement.

Bitewing mode

More sophisticated panoramic x-ray units include software functionality for acquiring bitewings. It should be noted that intraoral bitewings are still the gold standard. The physics of extraoral imaging techniques results in uneven magnification and reduction in the resolution of the image compared with intraoral images. However, in uncooperative patients, such as those with severe gagging reflexes, the bitewing mode on a panoramic unit may be an invaluable resource.

Dose reduction

Many factors determine the actual exposure dose to a patient and therefore make it difficult to compare one procedure directly with another. Exposure dose from a panoramic image is considered to be less than the cumulative exposure dose from a comparable full mouth series of intraoral x-ray images.

Cost effectiveness

A commonly used phrase is "time is money." In this case, an operator can perform the entire panoramic imaging procedure in as little as a few minutes with virtually no discomfort to the patient. Compare this to the much longer time required for an operator to generate a full set of intraoral x-ray images.

Standing position versus seated style panoramic unit

A standing position design of a panoramic x-ray unit offers three primary advantages over a seated version. (i) Seated patients often tend to hunch their back which produces a spinal shadow that can obscure a portion of the image. From personal experience, a standing position encourages patients to extend their necks straighter than when they are seated. The result will be a reduction in unwanted spinal shadows. (ii) The gantry can be lowered allowing physically handicapped patients in wheelchairs to remain in them for the entire procedure (Fig. M3). A wheelchair-bound patient simply needs to be wheeled into the

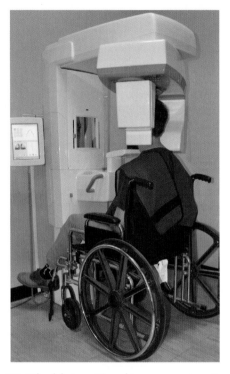

Fig. M3 Wheelchair positioned in a panoramic unit.

panoramic unit and the gantry can then be lowered around them. A sit-down panoramic unit requires physically transferring the patient from a wheelchair into the fixed panoramic chair. (iii) The footprint of a standing panoramic unit is smaller than a seated model, thus taking up less prime real estate space in a dental clinic.

Disadvantages

1. Diagnostic quality of a panoramic image is inferior to intraoral images
2. Distortion
3. Increased exposure to radiosensitive tissues
4. Misinterpretation
5. Equipment cost
6. Anatomic limitations

Diagnostic quality of a panoramic image is inferior to intraoral images

There are continued improvements occurring in panoramic digital technology. However, there are inherent principles of physics of extraoral imaging that are not encountered with intraoral imaging. As a result, the quality of a panoramic image remains inferior to intraoral images, although it is an excellent screening tool for assessing gross structures.

Distortion

Regardless of manufacturer, image magnification is unavoidable. Magnification will vary from one manufacturer's unit to another; ranging from 15% to 30%. In addition, errant patient positioning will produce uneven magnification within a panoramic image. The imaging software's measurement function cannot accurately account for the uneven magnification on panoramic images. Consequently, a numeric measure should only be considered as an estimate.

Increased exposure to radiosensitive tissues

Protective aprons with attached thyroid collars cannot be worn by patients during panoramic imaging. The protective collar will partially block the x-ray beam, resulting in a portion of the mandible being completely obscured on the panoramic image. As a result, sensitive regions of the neck cannot be protected from radiation exposure. Fortunately, the primary x-ray beam is highly collimated and a minimal amount of radiation reaches the thyroid region. In addition, minor amounts of internal scattering (i.e. x rays that bounce off the teeth and bones) may expose the thyroid gland. This is totally unavoidable.

Note: A double-sided protective apron that covers both the patient's front and back is recommended. During the exposure, the beam of radiation is directed from behind the patient. Therefore, a standard single-sided apron that covers only the front of the patient serves little benefit for panoramic imaging. Reversing it to cover the patient's back may be awkward as it may not remain in place.

Misinterpretation

Panoramic imaging also produces artifacts that can be misinterpreted, commonly referred to as "ghost images." A *ghost image* is a faint image of a radiodense object from one side of the patient that is superimposed onto the opposite side. A common example is earrings that are not removed prior to exposure. A faint radiopaque image of the right earring will be projected onto the left side and vice versa. Normal anatomic structures also produce ghost images. Regardless of the type of image being interpreted, the practitioner may misdiagnose normal from abnormal.

Equipment cost

The monetary cost of a panoramic x-ray unit is typically in the tens of thousands of dollars. Many different manufacturers market panoramic units with multiple features and varying costs. The practitioner should be an informed buyer as a panoramic x-ray unit should not need to be replaced for many years.

Anatomic limitations

A patient with *scoliosis* ♣♠ may not have adequate shoulder clearance for the panoramic unit to rotate unimpeded. A dry run without radiation should be attempted first to avoid unnecessarily exposing a patient to radiation. Alternatively, a full mouth series of intraoral images is recommended.

Technique errors

The following technical errors are discussed in this section:

1. Head is rotated or off-center
2. Head is positioned too far anterior (i.e. forward)
3. Head is positioned too far posterior (i.e. back)
4. Chin is tilted too far down
5. Chin is tilted up too high
6. Chin rest
7. Tongue position
8. Movement
9. Foreign objects
10. Protective (lead) apron

Head is rotated or off-center (Fig. M4)

Effect: If the dentition is positioned off-center, one side of the image will be magnified and the opposite side will be demagnified. The clinician should always compare the size of the teeth as well as the osseous structures bilaterally. Observing uniform differences in size from one side to the other should give the clinician pause to consider that it may simply be the result of an error in patient positioning.

   Solution: The operator should confirm that the mid-sagittal line is centered properly on the patient's face and that the back of the head is not positioned off-center. A patient can appear to be properly centered from the front but the back of the patient's head may be turned to one side.

Note: A clinical examination of the patient may reveal that the patient has a skeleto-dental deformity that will produce an asymmetric image.

Head is positioned too far anterior (i.e. forward) (Fig. M5)

Effect: If the dentition is positioned too far forward, the anterior teeth will be distorted, appearing constricted (i.e. narrowed) and the cervical vertebrae may be partially superimposed bilaterally over the rami and condyles.

   Solution: Ensuring that the patient's anterior teeth are biting properly onto the bite-block along with confirmation that the cuspid indicator is aligned properly should eliminate this problem. Patients should be guided by the operator into this position. Anteroposterior positioning errors may be inevitable if the patient has a *class II* or *class III occlusion* ☢.

Head is positioned too far posterior (i.e. back) (Fig. M6)

Effect: If the dentition is horizontally positioned too far back, the anterior teeth will be distorted, appearing magnified (i.e. widened) and the rami and condyles may be partially or wholly absent.

   Solution: Similar to when the patient's head is too far forward, the operator must ensure that the patient's anterior teeth are biting properly onto the bite-block and that the cuspid is properly aligned. Checking both of these alignments should eliminate this error. Patients should be guided by the operator into this position. Once again, positioning errors may be inevitable if the patient has a class II or III occlusion.

Chin is tilted too far down (Fig. M7)

Effect: If the dentition is tipped down too far, the *occlusal plane* ☢ will appear very steep. The steepness is dependent upon the amount of downward

Patient's right side

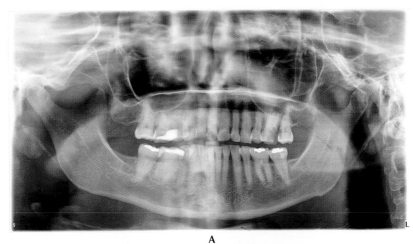

A

Patient's right side

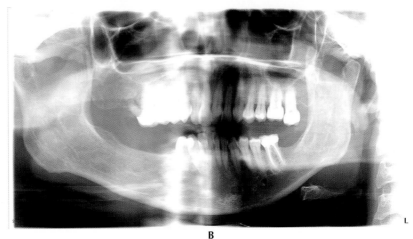

B

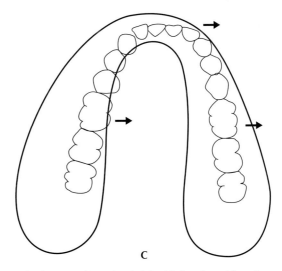

C

Fig. M4 A, B. Head positioned off-center. In both images the patient's right side is enlarged (i.e. distorted) compared to the left side. C. Illustration showing that dentition is off-centered.

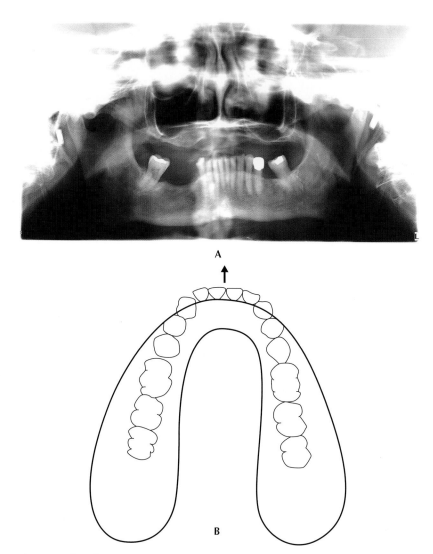

Fig. M5 A. Head positioned too far anteriorly. Note the spinal vertebrae encroaching from both sides and demagnification of the mandibular incisors. B. Illustration showing that dentition is too far forward.

tipping of the patient's head. The apices of the mandibular anterior teeth will invariably be out of focus as they will likely be positioned outside of the focal trough. Also, extreme downward tipping of the head may result in the condyles being projected off the superior aspect of the image.

Solution: Accurate head alignment using the Frankfort horizontal plane will eliminate this error. In so doing the operator should observe a small 5–7° downward tilt of the head.

Chin is tilted up too high (Fig. M8)

Effect: If the dentition is tipped up too high, the occlusal plane will appear very flat. The degree of flatness is dependent on the amount of upward tipping of the patient's head. The result is that the roots of the maxillary anterior teeth will invariably be out of focus as they will be positioned outside of the focal trough. Also, insufficient head tipping may result in the condyles being projected posteriorly off the posterior aspect of the image.

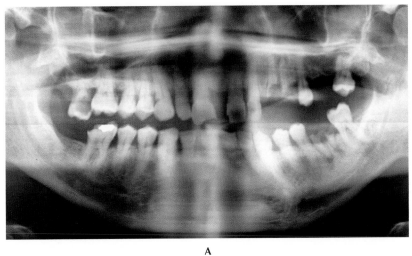

A

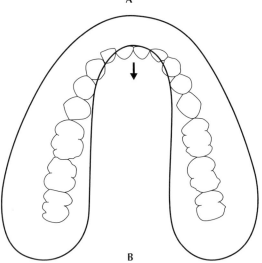

B

Fig. M6 A. Head positioned too far posteriorly. Note that the posterior aspect of the ramus is missing and magnification (i.e. widening) of the anterior maxillary and mandibular incisors. B. Illustration showing that dentition is too far back.

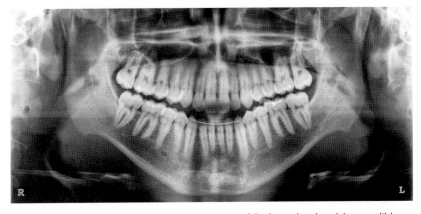

Fig. M7 Chin tilted down too far. Note the steep incline (V-shape) of the lower border of the mandible.

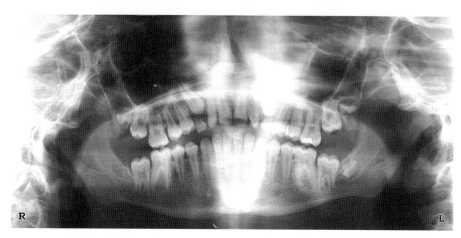

Fig. M8 Chin tilted up too high. Note the flat contour of the lower border of the mandible and the reverse *curve of Spee* ☢.

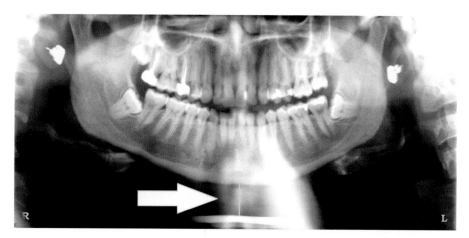

Fig. M9 Patient not positioned on chin rest. The yellow line indicates the gap beneath the chin and the chin rest.

Solution: As in the case above, accurate head alignment using the Frankfort horizontal plane is vital to prevent this error. Similarly, if the patient is in the proper position, the operator should observe a small 5–7° downward tilt of the head.

Chin rest (Fig. M9)

Effect: If the mandible is not seated onto the chin rest, the superior region encompassing the nasal fossa and maxillary sinuses will likely be partially cut off the top of the image while the region inferior to the submandibular region will be imaged. The region encompassing the dentition itself should not be affected.

Solution: Most panoramic units allow adjustment of the vertical height of the biteblock. The operator generally can slide the biteblock down to lower the patient's chin onto the chin rest.

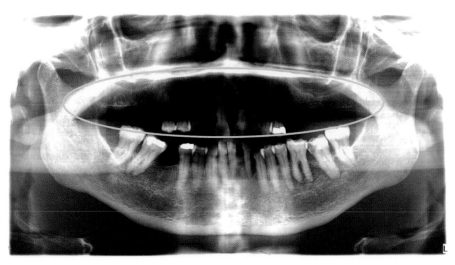

Fig. M10 Crescent-shaped radiolucent shadow produced by the palatoglossal air space (highlighted).

Tongue position (Fig. M10)

Effect: The tongue acts as a natural radiation filter and normally rests in the floor of the mouth. If the patient's tongue is allowed to remain at rest during a panoramic exposure, then a crescent-shaped radiolucent band will be produced that extends completely across the maxillary arch. This radiolucent band is the *palatoglossal air space* ☢. However, if a patient presses their tongue up against the palate, the tongue will absorb some of the excess radiation in the maxillary region and improve the overall diagnostic quality.

  Solution: The routine act of swallowing requires pressing one's tongue upward against the palate. For panoramic imaging, the operator should ask the patient to first swallow and then try to keep their tongue up against the roof of their mouth during the entire exposure.

Movement (Fig. M11)

Effect: A typical motion artifact will make the image appear wavy and disjointed. The operator should be aware that the source of radiation in a panoramic x-ray unit is collimated into a narrow vertical beam. The width of the x-ray beam is similar to the narrow light source that moves across a photocopier. Consequently only a small slice of the patient is actually exposed at any given time. If a patient moves momentarily, only the area exposed during that time of movement will be blurred (i.e. motion artifact), leaving the remainder of the image unaffected. Movement often occurs when one side of the panoramic unit contacts the patient's shoulder as it rotates around the patient. Reflexively the patient will move and lower their shoulder to permit the x-ray unit to pass by. Two physical contraindications that may cause motion artifacts are: (i) a short neck; and (ii) body tremor.

  Solution: When the operator suspects that there may not be adequate shoulder clearance for the x-ray unit to rotate around the patient because of a short neck, the operator should first do a test run without radiation. Panoramic machines typically have a test mode where there is no radiation output, yet the unit will still rotate normally. Performing a dry run avoids unnecessarily exposing a

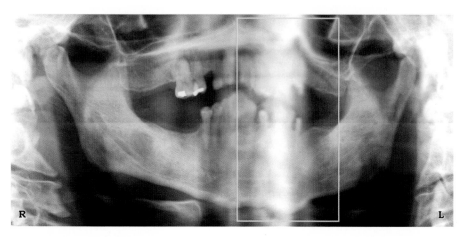

Fig. M11 Movement: the irregular contours of the patient's left side indicate patient movement during the exposure.

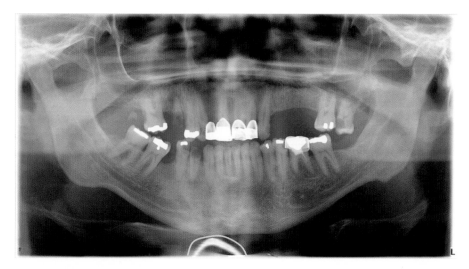

Fig. M12 Metallic necklace (highlighted).

patient to radiation. If the unit does rotate completely around unimpeded, then the operator should turn the radiation back on and repeat the procedure. For patients with a serious tremor, individual intraoral images are recommended as the exposure time for acquiring each image is very brief. Patient movement due to other reasons may not be predictable or avoidable.

Foreign objects (Figs M12 and M13)

Effect: Any foreign material can cast a radio-paque shadow on an image. The density of the resultant radiopacity is dependent upon the object's actual density and thickness. For panoramic imaging, the general rule is that metallic accessory items from the neckline upwards (e.g. necklaces, earrings, eyeglasses,

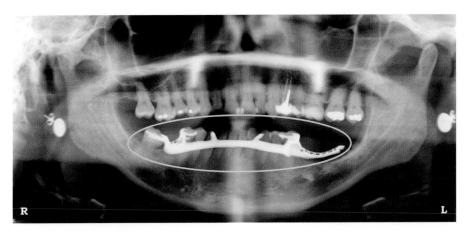

Fig. M13 Partial denture (highlighted).

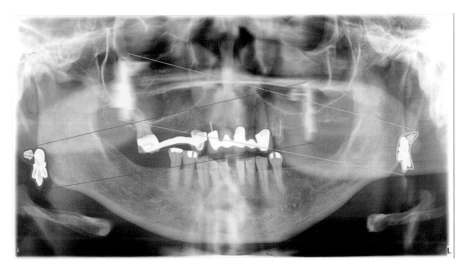

Fig. M14 Ghost images of right and left earrings (highlighted).

partial dentures) should be removed prior to the x-ray procedure. However, the operator must also be accepting of patients who may refuse or cannot easily remove various types of jewelry such as tongue bars, nose rings, etc. Any fixed dental restorations (e.g. crowns, fillings, permanent retainers) obviously cannot be removed. Partial dentures generally have metal clasps which will definitely obscure areas on an image. Therefore partial dentures should be

removed prior to taking a panoramic image. Any metal object will produce a *ghost image* ☢. A ghost image will be located slightly higher and on the opposite side to the object itself. The radiopacity of the ghost image is magnified and blurred compared with the causative object creating the ghost image (Figs M14 and M15).

Solution: As a routine, the operator at the outset should ask the patient to remove any jewelry worn from the neck up, including

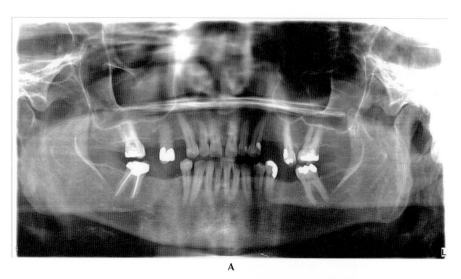

A

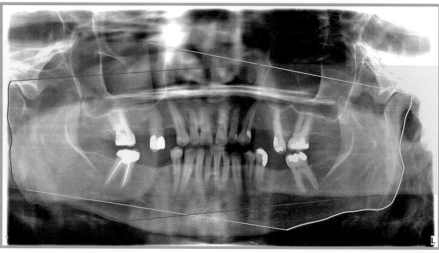

B

Fig. M15 Ghost images of right and left rami (highlighted in B).

eyewear and any removable dental prostheses. Hearing aids should remain in place until all of the instructions are given to the patient and then the patient should remove their hearing aid(s) for the actual procedure.

Note: An exception to this rule is a complete acrylic denture. Generally these will not be visible on an image and may be left in the patient's mouth to assist the operator when positioning the patient in the x-ray unit.

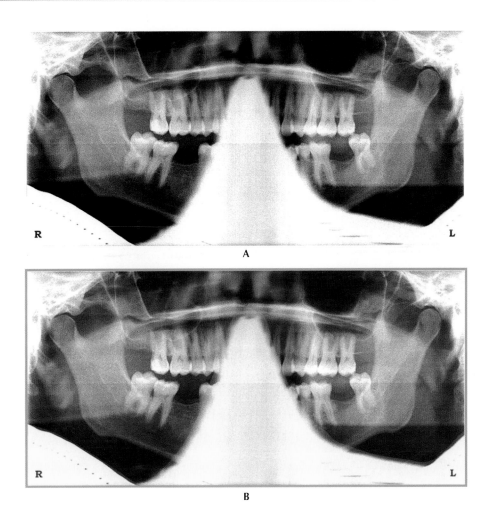

R A L

R B L

Fig. M16 Shadow of a thyroid collar worn during the procedure (highlighted in B).

Protective (lead) apron (Fig. M16)

Effect: The source of radiation in a panoramic unit is always directed from below the mandible. Consequently, if the protective apron has a thyroid collar attached, it will definitely be in the path of the x-ray beam. A dense, irregular-shaped radiopacity will appear in the midline–premolar area of the mandible.

Solution: If the apron has an attached thyroid collar, it must be removed or folded flat so as not to block the incoming path of the x-ray beam.

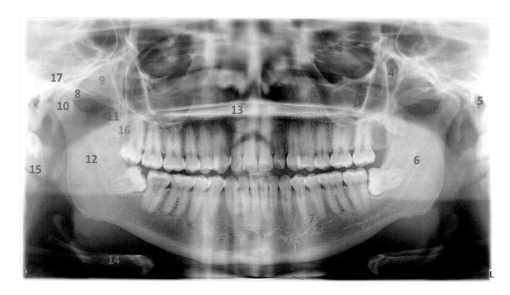

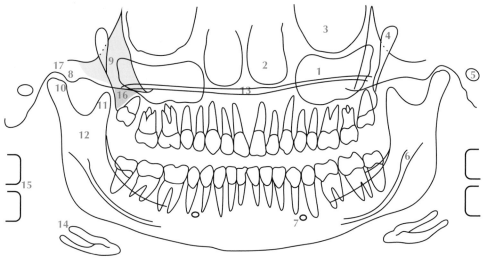

Fig. M17 Panoramic anatomy. See text for explanation of numbers 1 to 17.

Anatomic landmarks

Figure M17 shows the following landmarks:

1. Maxillary sinus
2. Nasal fossa
3. Orbit
4. Pterygomaxillary fissure
5. External auditory meatus
6. Mandibular canal
7. Mental foramen
8. Articular eminence
9. Zygoma (highlighted: yellow)
10. Condyle
11. Coronoid process
12. Ramus
13. Hard palate
14. Hyoid bone
15. Cervical vertebrae
16. Maxillary tuberosity (highlighted: orange)
17. Glenoid fossa

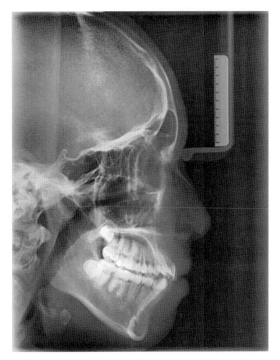

Fig. M18 Cephalograph image. (Source: Courtesy of Dr. Richard Ballard.)

2. LATERAL CEPHALOGRAPH IMAGING

A *lateral cephalograph* (aka lateral cephalogram or ceph) is a sagittal projection of the skull that includes both the hard and soft tissues (Fig. M18). The ability to visualize the soft tissue profile is essential when facial aesthetics are a concern, such as in orthodontic and oral surgical procedures. A cephalograph x-ray unit incorporates a head-holding device called a *cephalostat* ☢ (Fig. M19). Patient positioning requires gently inserting bilateral ear rods into the external auditory meatuses, a nasal rod positioned at the *nasion* ☢ and alignment of the Frankfort horizontal plane parallel to the floor (Fig. M20). In so doing, the patient's head is locked in place and affords the operator the ability to record the head position coordinates. In addition, it ensures proper alignment of the x-ray source with the

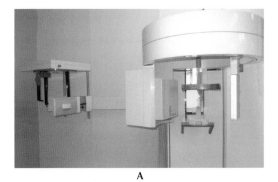

A

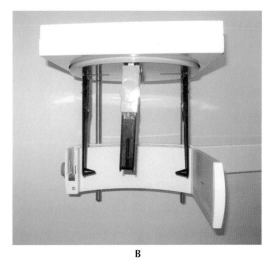

B

Fig. M19 A. Combined panoramic–cephalometric x-ray unit. B. Cephalostat attachment.

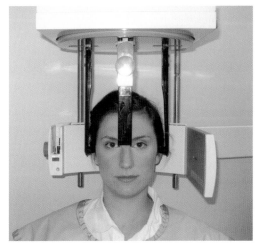

Fig. M20 Patient positioned in cephalostat.

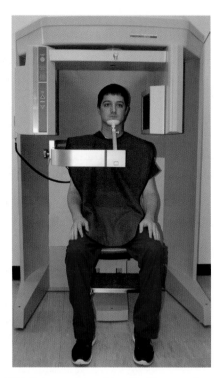

Fig. M21 Patient positioned in a CBCT x-ray unit.

imaging receptor. The positioning coordinates can be used to reproduce the original head alignment for follow-up imaging (e.g. monitor changes in growth and development). Typically, a cephalostat is an optional add-on arm attachment for most panoramic x-ray units, making it a combined panoramic–cephalometric unit. The combined x-ray unit shares the same x-ray source. The arm length is standardized at 152 cm and it is measured from the mid-sagittal plane of the patient's head to the x-ray source.

In comparison, a conventional lateral skull projection does not require a soft tissue filter nor does it require a cephalostat. At a minimum, a lateral skull projection requires a standard intraoral tubehead for the x-ray source and an appropriate-sized image receptor. The resultant image is a view of the osseous structures only (i.e. it lacks the soft tissue profile) and it is virtually impossible to accurately duplicate head position for follow-up images.

3. CONE BEAM COMPUTED TOMOGRAPHY

Introduction

Cone beam computed tomography (CBCT) ☢ technology was first developed for medicine in the 1980s. CBCT was introduced into the dental field in the late 1990s and has revolutionized dentistry ever since. Today, CBCT scanners are internationally manufactured in multiple configurations by numerous different companies (Fig. M21).

CBCT is a perfect example of how dental radiographic terminology is often self-explanatory. A CBCT x-ray unit generates a *beam* of x rays in the shape of a *cone*. Hundreds of individual x-ray images are rapidly exposed during the patient's scan. A *computer* algorithm combines the data to produce multiplanar *tomographic* ☢ images. The literal description is the technological term *"cone beam computed tomography."*

Depending upon the manufacturer's model, the patient may be in a seated, standing or supine position during the scan in any given CBCT x-ray unit. Most dental practices opt for a standing or seated version because the unit will occupy less floor space. In fact, a CBCT x-ray unit often physically resembles a conventional panoramic x-ray unit. However, unlike a panoramic unit where the *field of view (FOV)* ☢ is fixed for a given projection, CBCT x-ray units generally allow the operator to modify the width of the FOV. A flat panel receptor is typically used to capture the images. Maximum image size is dependent upon the size of the receptor. The vertical dimension (i.e. collimation height) is often the operator's primary consideration, while the horizontal dimension is usually secondary. For example, a large FOV cone beam x-ray unit may image up to 23 cm vertically, while a small FOV may only image 5 cm in a vertical dimension. In practice, a small FOV scan is ideal for endodontic procedures, single arch implants and most extraction cases. A large FOV scan is more practical for complex dual arch implant cases, complex oral surgery and orthodontic treatments. In general, a smaller volume of

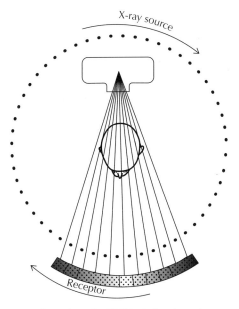

Fig. M22 Illustration of a CBCT tubehead rotating around the patient and exposing anywhere from 100 to several hundred individual images.

tissue imaged results in less overall radiation exposure dose to the patient and it also reduces the amount of *scatter radiation* ☢☢. Regardless of the size of the FOV, any radiation that deflects off metallic dental restorations, teeth and bones will diminish the overall image quality.

After following the manufacturer's patient positioning guidelines, it is usual for the operator to expose a preview or scout image prior to performing the actual scan. The purpose of the scout image is to confirm that the patient is positioned properly in the CBCT unit prior to performing the scan and for the operator to minimize the FOV to the region of interest. Unlike a panoramic unit, a CBCT gantry rotates a full 360° circle around the patient's head. A typical CBCT scan will expose between 100 and 600 individual lateral images sequentially as it rotates around the patient's head (Fig. M22). The scan acquisition time often is less than 10 s. Image data are characteristically captured using a *flat panel receptor* ☢☢. The preselected resolution for the scan will determine the total number of images exposed. A higher resolution scan will expose a greater number of individual

images allowing for thinner slice thicknesses compared with a lower resolution scan. From a technical standpoint, the only differences between a high resolution scan and a low resolution scan will be a slightly longer scan time and a longer reconstruction time because of the additional data collected. Regardless of resolution, complete reconstruction of the data is typically done within a few minutes. The clinician can selectively view the images in *axial* ☢☢, *sagittal* ☢☢ and *coronal* ☢☢ planes (Fig. M23).

How much radiation does a patient receive from a CBCT scan?

The radiation exposure dose of a CBCT scan is significantly higher than in conventional intraoral and extraoral dental imaging techniques and, as a result, a CBCT scan should not be used routinely on all patients. The National Council on Radiation Protection and Measurements (NCRP) has published CBCT guidelines and the American Academy of Oral and Maxillofacial Radiology has published position papers on CBCT for some of the dental specialties. Exposure doses from CBCT scans will vary significantly depending upon the volume size, image resolution, manufacturer specs, etc. According to the NCRP, the effective dose for a large FOV scan can be hundreds of microsieverts. For comparison, the effective dose of a typical digital panoramic image is approximately 15 μSv.

What is the legal responsibility of a clinician who orders a CBCT scan?

If the ordering clinician does not obtain an interpretive report from a radiologist, the clinician is responsible for diagnosing all pathology within the entire scan. It is extremely important to emphasize that this includes noting pathology located outside the area of interest. There are instances where CBCT scans needlessly use a maximum FOV for treatment planning a single mandibular implant. The clinician is still responsible for

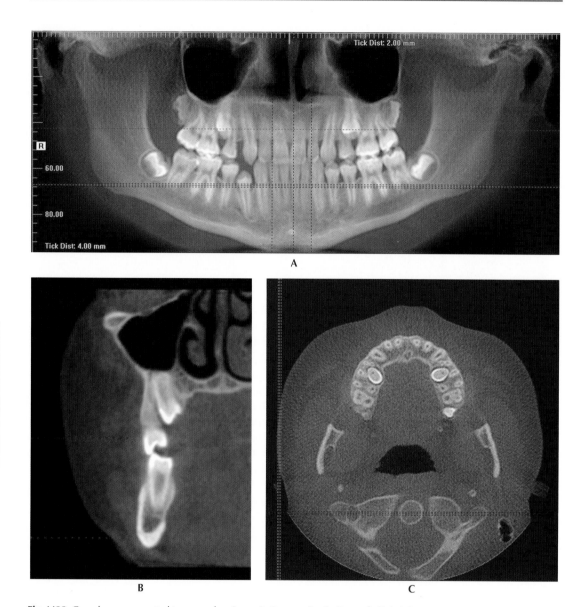

Fig. M23 Cone beam computed tomography views. A. Panoramic. B. Coronal. C. Axial.

identifying pathology located anywhere within the scan. Missed lesions could lead to legal consequences. This is a particular concern for clinicians who operate their own CBCT units and who may not seek outside services for an interpretive report.

Who should operate a CBCT x-ray unit?

Cone beam computed tomography imaging should only be performed by properly trained radiology personnel.

Should a CBCT unit be powered off at the end of the work day?

At the end of the day, similar to intraoral x-ray units, it is advisable to power down a CBCT x-ray unit to prolong the life of the x-ray tube contained within it. Unlike intraoral x-ray units, if the CBCT x-ray unit is turned off for an extended period of time, a warm-up period of approximately 30 min for the flat panel receptor is recommended prior to taking the first exposure. If the operator does not allow the unit adequate time to warm up to its proper operating temperature, then it may result in poorer quality images at the outset.

Anatomic landmarks

Figures M24 to M27 show the following landmarks.

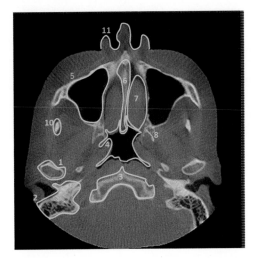

Fig. M24 Axial view: condylar level. See text for explanation of numbers 1 to 11.

Axial view: condylar level (Fig. M24)

1. Condylar head
2. Mastoid air cells
3. Cervical vertebra
4. Nasopharyngeal airway
5. Maxillary sinus
6. Nasal septum
7. Nasal concha
8. Lateral pterygoid plate
9. Medial pterygoid plate
10. Coronoid process
11. Soft tissue of the nose

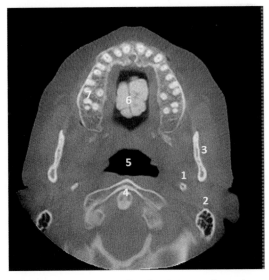

Fig. M25 Axial view: maxillary level. See text for explanation of numbers 1 to 7.

Axial view: maxillary level (Fig. M25)

1. Styloid process
2. Mastoid air cells
3. Ramus of the mandible
4. Cervical vertebra
5. Nasopharyngeal airway
6. Palatal torus
7. Maxillary arch

Axial view: mandibular level (Fig. M26)

1. Mandibular arch
2. Mandibular anterior teeth (i.e. roots of cuspids, lateral and central incisors)
3. Mandibular posterior teeth (i.e. roots of first and second molars)
4. Nasopharyngeal airway
5. Cervical vertebrae

Coronal view: molar region (Fig. M27)

1. Body of the mandible
2. Mental foramen
3. Mandibular second premolar
4. Palatoglossal airway space
5. Maxilla (palatine process)
6. Maxillary sinus
7. Nasal septum
8. Nasal concha
9. Tongue

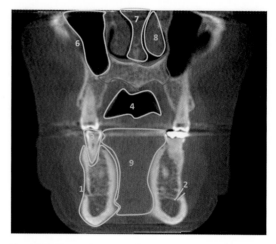

Fig. M27 Coronal view: molar region. See text for explanation of numbers 1 to 9.

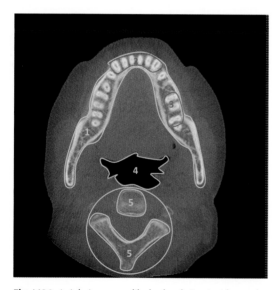

Fig. M26 Axial view: mandibular level. See text for explanation of numbers 1 to 5.

Applications

Cone beam computed tomography imaging should only be performed when conventional two-dimensional imaging is unable to adequately assess a patient's oral health or the outcome of a treatment. Regardless of the type of dental image projection prescribed (i.e. conventional or CBCT), the clinician must review the patient's history and perform a clinical examination first. The benefits to the patient should outweigh the potential risks of exposure to x rays and the minimum exposure necessary to achieve adequate image quality should be used.

The following applications will be discussed here:

1. Dental implants
2. Osseous pathology
3. Temporomandibular joint
4. Impactions
5. Orthodontics
6. Endodontics

Dental implants

Implants have become ubiquitous for tooth replacement today (Fig. M28). CBCT scans offer the practitioner invaluable pre- and post-surgical information. Some of the benefits include accurate localization of the inferior alveolar canal, cross-sectional visualization of the contours of the alveolar ridge and the ability to accurately measure the height and width of the alveolus. Additionally, fabrication of a surgical guide and use of pre-surgical treatment planning software provides the clinician invaluable information for assessing proper site selection and implant placement.

Osseous pathology

Three-dimensional views of osseous pathology can greatly assist treatment planning, particularly when oral surgery may be involved (Fig. M29). For example, bucco-lingual expansion of the mandibular ramus may be assessed from a CBCT scan which would be impossible to accurately view on a conventional two-dimensional panoramic image. Localization of anomalies such as a sialolith and a Stafne bone cyst can be diagnosed easily on sagittal and axial views.

Temporomandibular joint

Temporomandibular joint dysfunction (TMD) may be related to osseous changes ongoing in the temporomandibular joint. CBCT imaging of the temporomandibular joint is excellent for revealing degenerative and neoplastic changes in the region (Figs M30 and M31).

(a)

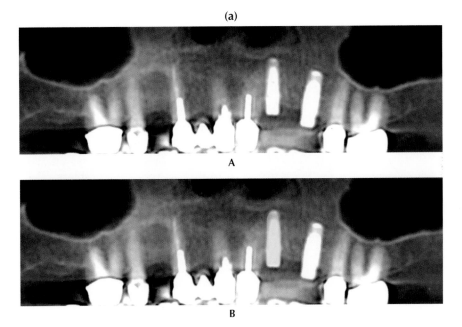

A

B

Fig. M28 **(a)** Post-implant placement of implants no. 10 (highlighted in B) and no. 12; both appear well-positioned.

(b)

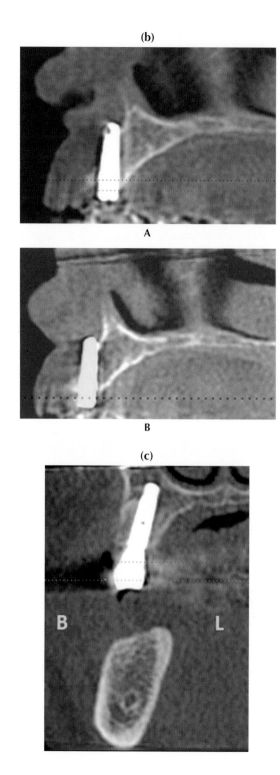

A

B

(c)

B   L

Fig. M28 (Continued) **(b)** Cross-sectional image revealing that implant no. 10 has clearly perforated through the labial cortical plate. The surgical error was not visible on the panoramic view. **(c)** Properly positioned implant within the confines of the cortical plates. B, buccal side; L, lingual side.

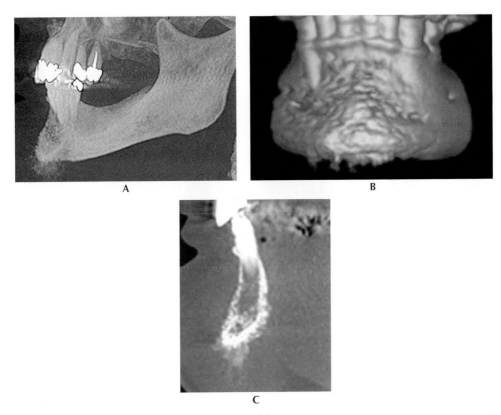

Fig. M29 Osteosarcoma with classic *sunburst appearance* ☢ of the anterior aspect of the mandible. A. Lateral view. B. Three-dimensional rendering of the afflicted area. C. Cross-sectional view.

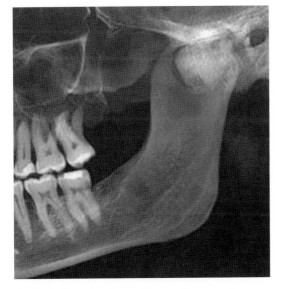

Fig. M30 Osteochondroma. (Source: Courtesy of Dr. G. Klasser.)

Impaction

Three-dimensional CBCT images revealing tooth to tooth and tooth to anatomic structures relationships can be invaluable. Clinicians performing a routine dental extraction may not benefit from a CBCT scan. However, a CBCT image could be beneficial for localizing impacted teeth. Extractions of impacted mandibular third molars often are complicated by their proximity to the inferior alveolar canal. Relying on a conventional two-dimensional panoramic image or intraoral periapical image may inadequately relate the impacted tooth to the canal. Cross-sectional views will more accurately relate the positions of the two objects to one another (Fig. M32). In addition, the clinician will obtain supplemental information as to whether a buccal or lingual approach would be best to access the tooth.

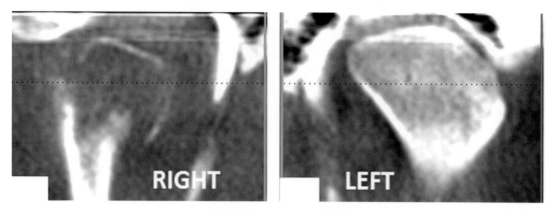

Fig. M31 Coronal view of metastatic carcinoma affecting the right condyle versus an unaffected condyle on the image labeled "left."

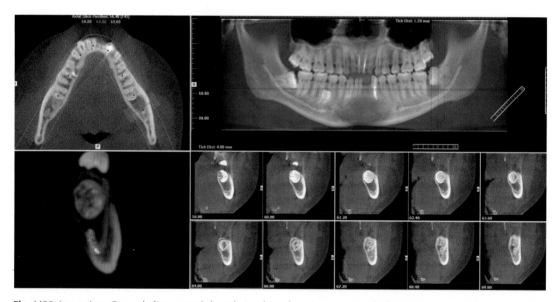

Fig. M32 Impaction. Coronal slices reveal the relationship of crown no. 17 with the unilocular radiolucency and the mandibular canal (highlighted)

Orthodontics

Cone beam computed tomography imaging can supplement cephalographic and panoramic images for treatment planning (Fig. M33), but it should not be standard protocol for all patients. A CBCT scan is particularly useful when it may be impossible for a clinician to visualize the positional relationships of unerupted teeth using two-dimensional conventional images. Multiplanar images from CBCT scans will supply the clinician much more detailed relational information critical to the treatment.

Endodontics

Cone beam computed tomography imaging is useful for locating accessory canals, fractures and localization of apical pathology. For example, a periapical image may reveal a radiolucent lesion that appears to envelope multiple roots. However, a cross-sectional image may reveal

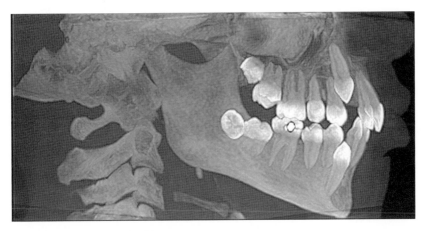

Fig. M33 Cephalograph reconstruction (CBCT).

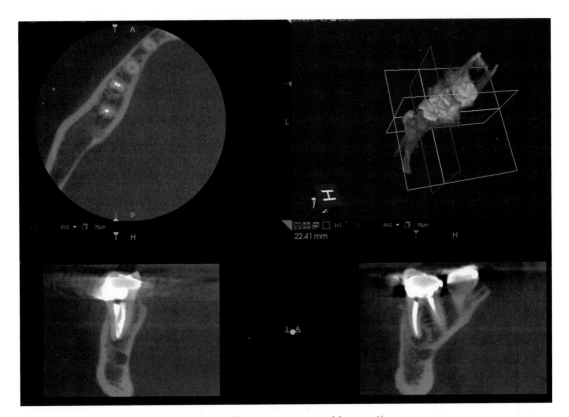

Fig. M34 Small field of view resulting in reduced patient exposure and fewer artifacts.

that the radiolucency is actually attached to only a single root which will then alter the treatment. CBCT x-ray units designed to image a single quadrant with a small FOV (e.g. 5 cm) is ideally suited for endodontic procedures (Fig. M34). It reduces overall scatter radiation and exposes the patient to significantly less radiation compared with other scans.

Quality Assurance

"Quality assurance" (QA) is defined in the Merriam-Webster dictionary as a program for the systematic monitoring and evaluation of the various aspects of a service or a facility to ensure that standards of quality are being met. Radiologic quality assurance in a dental practice refers to the proper functioning of all x-ray equipment to acquire optimum diagnostic images with minimal radiation exposure to the patient, dental office personnel and the general public. Radiation safety within a dental office is the responsibility of the dentist.

All x-ray machines must be periodically inspected for QA either by a state radiation safety inspector or by a private dental service company. There are simple and relatively inexpensive testing procedures that are used to identify problems with all forms of dental x-ray equipment. These tests and the subsequent corrections must be performed to avoid subjecting a patient to unnecessary radiation exposure. QA also helps to improve the diagnostic quality of the resultant x-ray images. Inspectors will measure the consistency and quantity of radiation output from each x-ray unit, analyze the collimation and alignment of the beam of radiation and test the accuracy and reproducibility of the exposure timer. All x-ray equipment sold in the United States must meet minimum beam filtration standards and therefore is unlikely to need correction. For extraoral units such as panoramic x-ray units, measurements of the slit beam will also be necessary.

Fundamentals of Oral and Maxillofacial Radiology, First Edition. J. Sean Hubar.
© 2017 John Wiley & Sons, Inc. Published 2017 by John Wiley & Sons, Inc.
Companion website: www.wiley.com/go/hubar/radiology

O Infection Control

Universal infection control guidelines must be followed by all dental personnel to protect cross-contamination between patients and between patients and dental healthcare workers. After the recognition of AIDS in the 1980s, infection control procedures became prioritized. Some of the other more common transmissible infections include hepatitis, tuberculosis and herpes. These guidelines are necessary to protect all individuals from exposure to disease spread by blood and bodily fluids. Both the American Dental Association (ADA) and the Centers for Disease Control and Prevention (CDC) recommend *universal precautions* ☢ for everyone as many patients may fail to report their illnesses to the dentist or may not even be aware that they are infected at the time of their appointment. The placement of receptors intraorally by an operator and then the handling of the tubehead and control panel results in numerous avenues for cross-contamination to occur in a dental operatory while performing routine imaging procedures.

Excerpt from "CDC Guidelines for Infection Control in Dental Health-Care Settings"

When taking radiographs, the potential to cross-contaminate equipment and environmental surfaces with blood or saliva is high if aseptic technique is not practiced. Gloves should be worn when taking radiographs and handling contaminated film packets. Other PPE (e.g. mask, protective eyewear, and gowns) should be used if spattering of blood or other body fluids is likely. Heat-tolerant versions of intraoral radiograph accessories are available and these semi-critical items (e.g. film holding and positioning devices) should be heat sterilized before patient use.

Protective barriers should be used, or any surfaces that become contaminated should be cleaned and disinfected with an EPA registered hospital disinfectant of low- (HIV and HBV claim) to intermediate-level (tuberculocidal claim) activity. Radiography equipment (e.g. radiograph tubehead and control panel) should be protected with surface barriers that are changed after each patient. If barriers are not used, equipment that has come into contact with DHCP's gloved hands should be cleaned and then disinfected after each patient use.

Digital radiography receptors and other high-technology instruments (e.g. intraoral camera, electronic periodontal probe, occlusal analyzers, and lasers) come into contact with mucous membranes and are considered semi-critical devices. They should be cleaned and ideally heat-sterilized for high level disinfection between patients. However, these items vary by manufacturer or type of device in their ability to be sterilized or high-level disinfected. Semi-critical items that cannot be reprocessed by heat sterilization or high-level disinfection should, at a minimum, be barrier protected by using an FDA cleared barrier to reduce gross contamination during use. Use of a barrier does not always protect from contamination. One study determined that a brand of commercially available plastic barriers used to protect dental digital radiography receptors failed at a substantial rate (44%). This rate dropped to 6% when latex finger cots were used in conjunction with the plastic

Fundamentals of Oral and Maxillofacial Radiology, First Edition. J. Sean Hubar.
© 2017 John Wiley & Sons, Inc. Published 2017 by John Wiley & Sons, Inc.
Companion website: www.wiley.com/go/hubar/radiology

barrier. To minimize the potential for device-associated infections, after removing the barrier, the device should be cleaned and disinfected with an EPA registered hospital disinfectant (intermediate-level) after each patient. Manufacturers should be consulted regarding appropriate barrier and disinfection/sterilization procedures for digital radiography receptors, other high technology intraoral devices and computer components.

Source: Kohn *et al.* (2003)

All dental personnel directly involved with patient care must wear protective clothing (Fig. O1). Disposable or non-disposable gowns must be long-sleeved, at least three-quarter in length, and have a closed collar. In addition, disposable protective gloves should always be worn by the operator during receptor and tubehead placement to minimize risks to the operator and patient. It is recommended that gloves not be put on until after the patient is seated in the operatory. After seating the patient, it is recommended that the operator first wash their hands and then glove up in full view of the patient. Gloving up in front of the patient assures the patient that the operator's gloves are fresh, not having been worn

whilst treating a prior patient. Similarly, all x-ray instrumentation should be unpackaged in open view of the patient to reassure the patient that everything is sterile. For intraoral and extraoral imaging procedures, aerosols are not generated but exposure to bodily fluids is still unavoidable. Consequently, operators may also wish to wear protective eyewear and a mask or face shield. Image receptors must be covered with disposable plastic non-permeable wraps (Fig. O2).

General instructions for cleaning and disinfecting a solid-state receptor (courtesy of Sirona™)

Unless the manufacturer states differently, the cable should remain attached to the receptor. Similarly, for wireless receptors, the battery pack should be removed from the receptor and cleaned separately, following the same steps as the receptor. Exercise care when cleaning around the battery contacts to avoid damaging them.

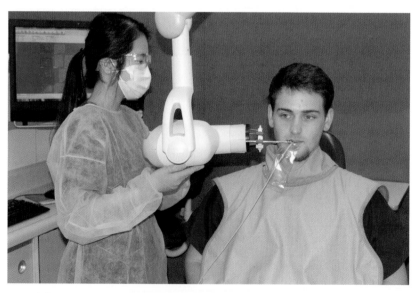

Fig. O1 Operator in full infection control compliance: wearing a long sleeve gown, disposable gloves, face mask and protective eyewear. The patient is wearing a protective apron with thyroid collar.

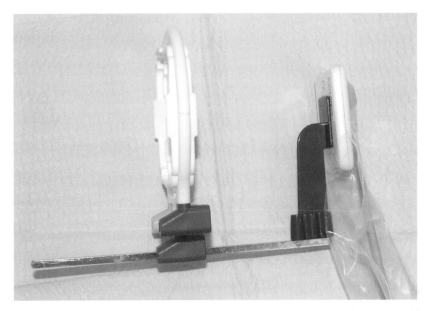

Fig. O2 Intraoral receptor holder attached to a direct dental receptor inside a protective infection control barrier cover.

Before using a receptor the first time and before every new patient, the following protocol is recommended:

1. Remove and discard all protective hygienic barriers and/or sheaths from the receptor prior to removing disposable gloves.
2. Place the receptor on a tray covered by a disposable liner, or in a receptacle that can be thoroughly disinfected.
3. Remove and discard gloves.
4. Wash hands and put on a new pair of disposable gloves.
5. Disconnect the receptor from the remote module.
6. If the receptor or cable are visibly soiled (e.g. blood or saliva contamination), each should be cleaned with a soapy cloth or paper towel, and then dried with a clean lint-free cloth or paper towel.
7. Thoroughly wipe the receptor and cable (if applicable) with a disinfecting product. Do not expose the contacts of the receptor/remote module connection to liquid.
8. Repeat step 7. When the receptor has been wiped two times, continue with the following steps.
9. Remove potential chemical build-up from the receptor by wiping it with a sterile lap sponge saturated with de-ionized water.
10. Use a sterile dry lap sponge to dry the receptor or cable, as needed.
11. Place the receptor in a clean environment, ready for next use.
12. Reconnect the receptor.
13. Remove and card gloves.

P

Occupational Radiation Exposure Monitoring

Who should be monitored?

Occupational Safety and Health Administration (OSHA) regulations state that anyone who is occupationally exposed to x rays and could potentially receive more than 25% of the quarterly occupational dose limit, are required to wear a dosimeter (29 CFR 1910.1096(d)(2)(i)). The NCRP (1998) recommends that all personnel who are likely to receive an effective dose greater than 1 mSv per year be monitored. If an operator follows normal radiation safety precautions (i.e. avoid being in the primary beam, standing at least 2 m from the source or behind a barrier, etc.) the number of dental workers who exceed this dose will be very few.

How is radiation exposure monitored?

A personal dosimetry badge is worn by dental personnel for recording cumulative x-radiation dose in the workplace (see Fig. G10). After a specified period of time, the badge must be returned to the monitoring service provider for reading. The time interval can vary (e.g. 1 week, 1 month, 3 months, etc.). Three months is a practical time interval for many dental offices (exception: see question about pregnant worker). A written report for each dosimeter will be issued by the monitoring provider.

Who monitors dental radiation exposure?

A number of different companies offer monitoring services for dental office personnel. A nominal fee is charged for each radiation dosimetry badge.

Why should office personnel be monitored?

All ionizing radiation is harmful.

What happens if my radiation exposure report exceeds the maximum exposure dose permitted?

If a radiation badge records a dose in excess of that recommended by either the OSHA or the NCRP, the individual involved must be

Fundamentals of Oral and Maxillofacial Radiology, First Edition. J. Sean Hubar.
© 2017 John Wiley & Sons, Inc. Published 2017 by John Wiley & Sons, Inc.
Companion website: www.wiley.com/go/hubar/radiology

informed about the dose and an investigation will need to be undertaken to determine the cause. The individual may be temporarily prohibited from working around x-ray equipment. The dosimetry results are taken very seriously by OSHA, so fellow co-workers should not play pranks by removing another employee's badge and intentionally exposing it to radiation.

How is a pregnant employee monitored for radiation exposure?

In addition to the standard radiation badge, a supplemental fetal radiation badge should be worn for monitoring radiation dose to the fetus over the term of the pregnancy. A pregnant employee should be monitored on a monthly basis for the term of the pregnancy.

I work at the front desk away from the dental x-ray unit. Why should I be monitored?

All personnel should be monitored for a minimum of 1 year to ensure that the readings do not exceed the minimum set by the OSHA and NCRP. This includes front desk receptionists, business managers and laboratory technicians within the dental office.

How long do I need to be monitored?

For new or relocated x-ray equipment, the proprietor shall provide personal radiation badges for at least 1 year to assess and document doses to all personnel. However, if the work environment changes regarding x-ray exposure for that employee, then monitoring should be reinstituted for another period of time until the radiation exposure levels are reported to be negligible. New operators of hand-held x-ray units should be monitored for 1 year. If the dosimetry badge reports repeatedly show negligible exposure, the proprietor may decide to discontinue monitoring after 1 year (see question about pregnant worker).

How long should the office keep radiation exposure records?

Records should be kept permanently. This protects the dental proprietor from possible future litigation. A former employee years later may develop an illness that he or she may attempt to link back to employment in the dental office as the root cause. A dosimetry report would be a beneficial piece of evidence to help exonerate the dentist in this situation.

When should radiation badges not be worn?

A radiation badge is not to be worn when the wearer is subjected to diagnostic exposures as a patient and it should not be worn outside the dental office. Whenever a radiation badge is not worn, it should be stored in a radiation-safe area. Tampering with or use of radiation badges for any purposes other than those intended cannot be condoned.

Q Hand-held X-ray Systems

Portable x-ray units for commercial use have been manufactured for many decades. The Fexitron 845 was a portable x-ray generator manufactured by the Field Emission Corporation (McMinnville, OR) in the 1960s. This unit was bulky, heavy and unsuitable for intraoral imaging. Today many companies manufacture hand-held intraoral x-ray units. They are small, lightweight and often resemble a cordless power drill (Fig. Q1). Contrary to a traditional wall-mounted x-ray unit where the operator can be protected by distance and physical barriers, a well-designed hand-held system must incorporate additional shielding to minimize the dose to the hands and body of the operator.

Dental radiographic examinations: recommendations for patient selection and limiting radiation exposure

Hand-held, battery-powered x-ray systems are available for intra-oral radiographic imaging. The hand-held exposure device is activated by a trigger on the handle of the device. However, dosimetry studies indicate that these hand-held devices present no greater radiation risk than standard dental radiographic units to the patient or the operator. No additional radiation protection precautions are needed when the device is used according to the manufacturer's instructions. These include: 1. holding the device at mid-torso height, 2. orienting the shielding ring properly with respect to the operator, and 3. keeping the cone as close to the patient's face as practical. If the hand-held device is operated without the ring shield in place, it is recommended that the operator wear a lead apron.

All operators of hand-held units should be instructed on their proper storage. Due to the portable nature of these devices, they should be secured properly when not in use to prevent accidental damage, theft, or operation by an unauthorized user. Hand-held units should be stored in locked cabinets, locked storage rooms, or locked work areas when not under the direct supervision of an individual authorized to use them. Units with user-removable batteries should be stored with the batteries removed. Records listing the names of approved individuals who are granted access and use privileges should be prepared and kept current.

Source: American Dental Association (2012)

Commentary

There are several scenarios in which the use of a hand-held x-ray unit is advantageous. Examples include treating patients in confined spaces such as a mobile dental clinic, patients under sedation who are unresponsive and for operators conducting forensic work at disaster sites. For all of these situations, it would either be impractical or impossible to use a fixed dental x-ray unit.

Fundamentals of Oral and Maxillofacial Radiology, First Edition. J. Sean Hubar.
© 2017 John Wiley & Sons, Inc. Published 2017 by John Wiley & Sons, Inc.
Companion website: www.wiley.com/go/hubar/radiology

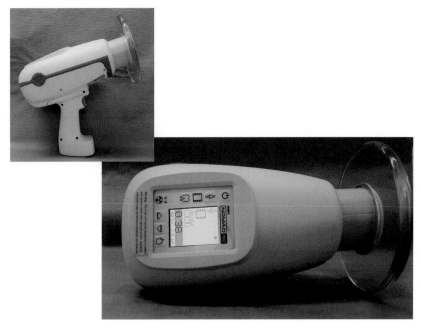

Fig. Q1 NOMAD Pro™ hand-held (portable) x-ray unit.

The NCRP and the ADA both condone the use of hand-held x-ray units. However it is the opinion of this author that because of unknown risks associated with repeated low doses of radiation to the operator, dental offices should continue to use fixed x-ray units. Fixed dental x-ray units result in lower radiation exposure to the operator by using remote activation (i.e. operator standing outside the operatory during the exposure). A fixed unit also offers greater flexibility in selecting exposure settings which can produce a better diagnostic image. Whenever it is possible, the operator should use a fixed dental x-ray unit.

Part Two Interpretation

R Localization of Objects (SLOB Rule)

Standard intraoral periapical and bitewing images only offer two-dimensional anterior–posterior and superior–inferior perspectives. Localization of foreign objects and impacted teeth, differentiating a buccal versus lingual canal in a single root during endodontic procedures, etc. all require a bucco-lingual perspective. An occlusal image taken in conjunction with routine periapical and bitewing images can possibly offer the practitioner such a bucco-lingual perspective. Superimposition of anatomic structures and distortion of the image are both inherent problems with the occlusal technique that often obfuscate the image.

In lieu of using CBCT imaging, an alternative intraoral technique for object localization is the *tube-shift method*. It goes by different terms, including *Clark's* rule, the *buccal object* rule and the *SLOB* rule. "SLOB" is an acronym for **s**ame–**l**ingual, **o**pposite–**b**uccal. C. A. Clark first described this technique back in 1909, thus the eponym "Clark's rule." This should not be confused with the unrelated medical term, *Clark's rule,* which is a formula to calculate medicine dosage for children.

The principle of the tube-shift technique simply requires exposing two different angulated intraoral x-ray images of one area. The first image acts as a reference image. The horizontal or vertical angulation of the PID is then modified prior to taking a second image of the same area (Figs R1 and R2). Comparison of the two images for positional changes of the object of interest will determine if it is located more towards the buccal or lingual aspect. For example, if the PID is horizontally shifted mesially in comparison to the first image and the object in question appears to move distally (i.e. in the opposite direction to the PID), the object of interest is positioned on the buccal side. If the object of interest moves in the same direction as the PID, then the object is positioned towards the lingual side. Conversely, if the PID is horizontally shifted distally in comparison to the first image and the object moves mesially, the object of interest is positioned on the buccal.

The same principle applies in a vertical shift mode. For example, if the PID is shifted superiorly in comparison to the reference image and the object in question appears to move inferiorly (i.e. in the opposite direction to the PID), the object of interest is positioned on the buccal side. If the object of interest moves in the same direction as the PID, then the object is positioned more towards the lingual side. Conversely, if the PID is shifted inferiorly in

Fundamentals of Oral and Maxillofacial Radiology, First Edition. J. Sean Hubar.
© 2017 John Wiley & Sons, Inc. Published 2017 by John Wiley & Sons, Inc.
Companion website: www.wiley.com/go/hubar/radiology

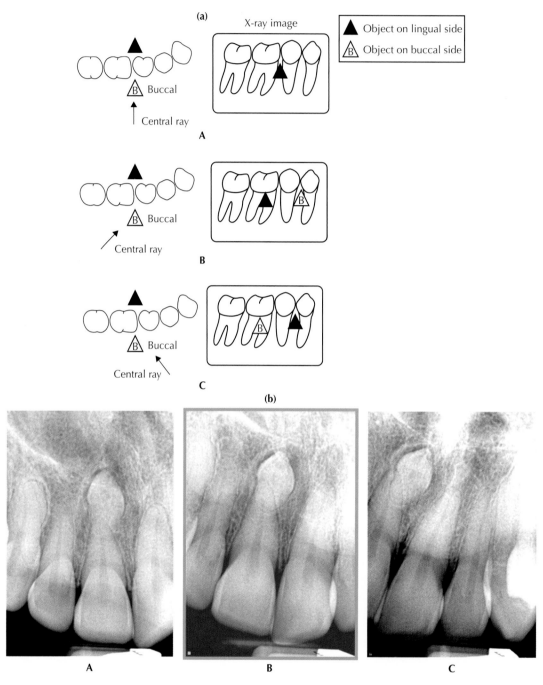

Fig. R1 **(a)** Illustration of the SLOB rule: horizontal angulation shift of the PID. A. Central ray directed perpendicular to the receptor superimposes both objects (▲ ⊿). B. Central ray directed from posterior position projects ⊿ anteriorly (i.e. opposite direction). C. Central ray directed from the anterior position projects ⊿ posteriorly (i.e. opposite direction). Conclusion: ⊿ is on the buccal and ▲ is on the lingual. **(b)** A. Central lateral view (nos 7 and 8). B. Horizontal shift of the PID (nos 8 and 9) resulted in a shift of the mesiodens to the patient's left. C. Further horizontal shift of the PID (nos 9 and 10) resulted in a further shift of the mesiodens in the same direction. Conclusion: the mesiodens is on the lingual aspect.

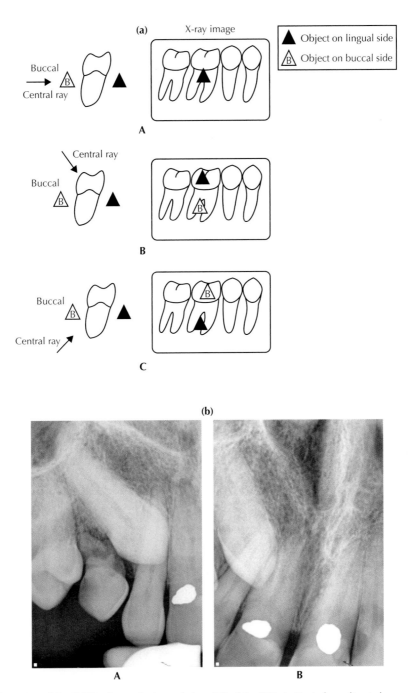

Fig. R2 (a) Illustration of the SLOB rule: vertical angulation shift of the PID. A. Central ray directed perpendicular to the receptor superimposes both objects (▲ ⚠). B. Central ray directed from superior position projects ⚠ inferiorly (i.e. opposite direction). C. Central ray directed from the inferior position projects ⚠ superiorly (i.e. opposite direction). Conclusion: ⚠ is on the buccal and ▲ is on the lingual. **(b)** A. Central lateral view (nos 7 and 8). B. Increased vertical angulation resulted in a shift of the unerupted cuspid superiorly (same direction as the PID movement). Simultaneously, a horizontal shift of the PID to the midline resulted in a shift of the cuspid toward the midline (same direction as the PID). Conclusion: the cuspid is on the lingual aspect.

comparison to the first image and the object in question appears to move superiorly, the object of interest is positioned on the buccal. If the object of interest moves in the same direction as the PID, then the object is positioned more towards the lingual.

In situations where a foreign object is located in an edentulous region, the practitioner may still be able to apply the SLOB rule simply by utilizing dental anatomic landmarks as a guide. In this scenario, one must study the position of the object in relation to a reference landmark. If the object moves either away from the landmark or in the same direction as the landmark, its position can be determined within either jaw. Similarly, when multiple images have already been exposed as in a full mouth series of images, the practitioner should focus on specific landmarks to determine an alteration in either the horizontal or vertical position to localize an object. In either case, the practitioner should first attempt to use pre-existing images for diagnosis prior to pre-scribing additional images.

S Recommendations for Interpreting Images

Interpretation of dental x-ray images is integral to oral diagnosis and treatment planning. The best technology cannot correct for visual miscues. When examining x-ray images, dental professionals all too often focus solely on the teeth and fail to see alterations to the surrounding structures, unless, of course, they are too obvious to miss. The accompanying panoramic image outlines multiple anatomic structures (Fig. S1). In any order, the observer should systematically evaluate each structure or pair of structures independently: the maxillary sinuses, the orbits, the border of the mandible, the temporomandibular joint, the border of the maxilla, the dentition, etc. Doing so will reduce the number of anomalies missed. The author's recommendation is for the observer to consistently use one sequential visual pattern and simply adapt it for each type of image viewed (i.e. intraoral, panoramic, cephalometric and CBCT images). It is also recommended that evaluation of the teeth and large osseous lesions be diagnosed toward the end of the interpretation. At that time, the observer can solely focus on alterations to the dentition and include large osseous anomalies. This should improve the diagnostic proficiency of the clinician.

Fundamentals of Oral and Maxillofacial Radiology, First Edition. J. Sean Hubar.
© 2017 John Wiley & Sons, Inc. Published 2017 by John Wiley & Sons, Inc.
Companion website: www.wiley.com/go/hubar/radiology

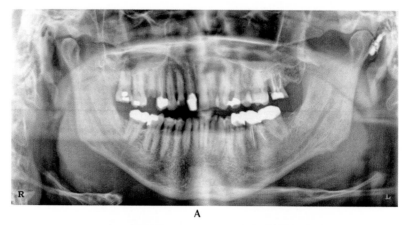

A

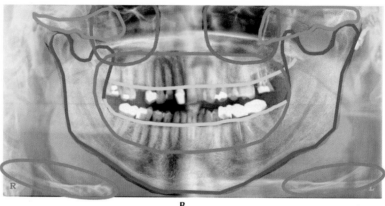

B

Fig. S1 Interpretation of a panoramic image. Red, maxillary sinuses; purple, mandible; yellow line, maxilla; green, zygomatic arch; magenta, hyoid bone; yellow shading, surrounding structures; blue, dentition.

Systematic observation order:

1. Red: maxillary sinuses (right and left)
2. Purple: mandible (exclude the teeth)
3. Yellow line: alveolar crestal bone, both maxilla and mandible
4. Green: zygomatic arch
5. Magenta: hyoid bone
6. Yellow shading: surrounding structures
7. Blue: maxillary and mandibular teeth

X-ray Puzzles: Spot the Differences

The following section contains eight pairs of extraoral dental images. The object of this exercise is for the observer to locate subtle differences between two near-identical x-ray images. The changes are highlighted in the accompanying image. The intent of the author is to demonstrate that a thorough analysis of every image is critical to find all of the anomalies. Hopefully these puzzles and the interpretation recommendations previously mentioned will help train the observer to more critically examine every x-ray image and become a better diagnostician.

Fundamentals of Oral and Maxillofacial Radiology, First Edition. J. Sean Hubar.
© 2017 John Wiley & Sons, Inc. Published 2017 by John Wiley & Sons, Inc.
Companion website: www.wiley.com/go/hubar/radiology

Puzzle 1

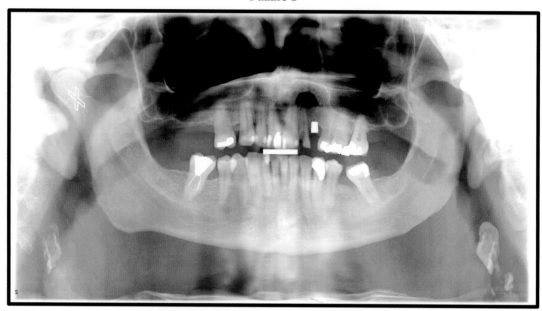

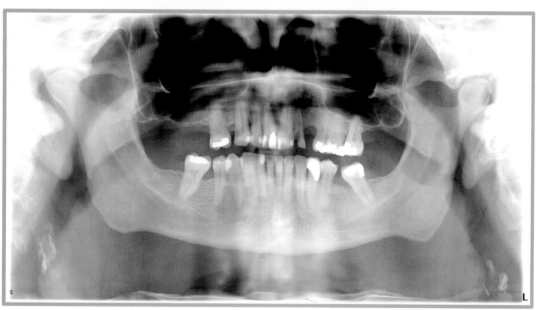

Spot ten differences between the panoramic images
Please see page 122 for solution

Puzzle 2

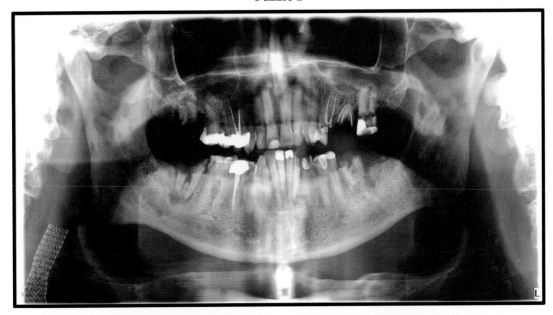

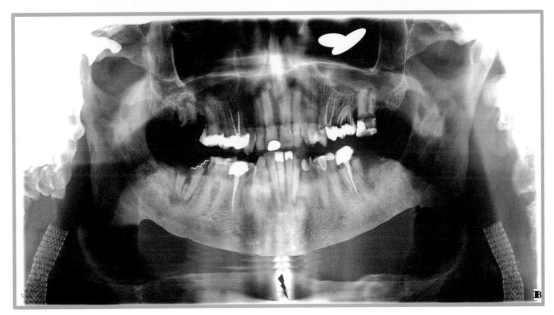

Spot ten differences between the panoramic images
Please see page 122 for solution

Puzzle 3

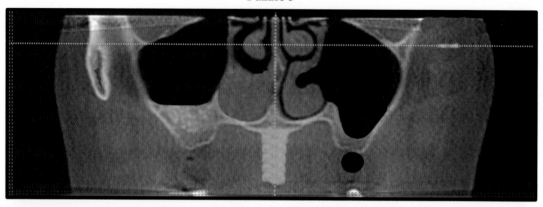

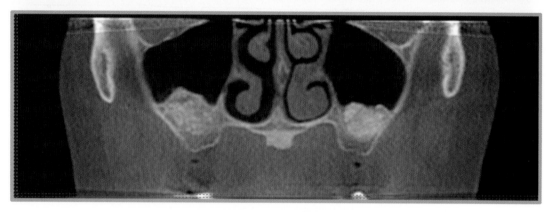

Spot ten differences between the coronal images
Please see page 122 for solution

Puzzle 4

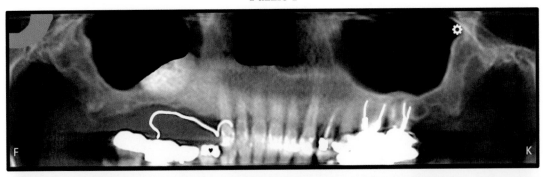

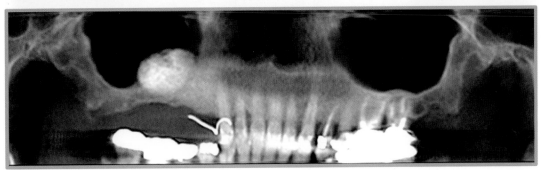

Spot ten differences between the coronal images
Please see page 122 for solution

Puzzle 5

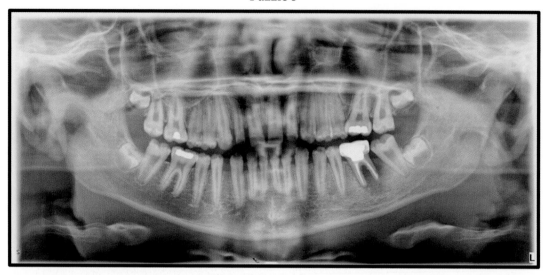

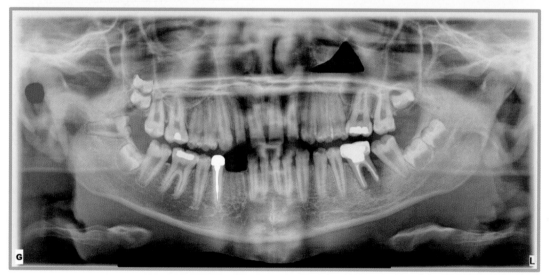

Spot nine differences between the panoramic images
Please see page 123 for solution

Puzzle 6

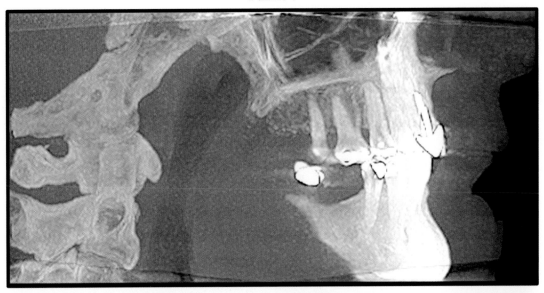

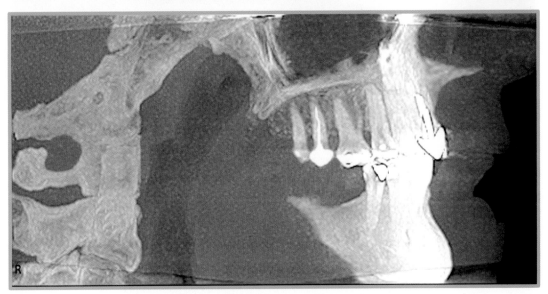

Spot nine differences between the mid-sagittal images
Please see page 123 for solution

Puzzle 7

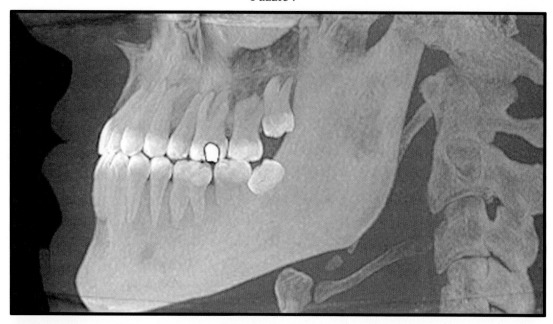

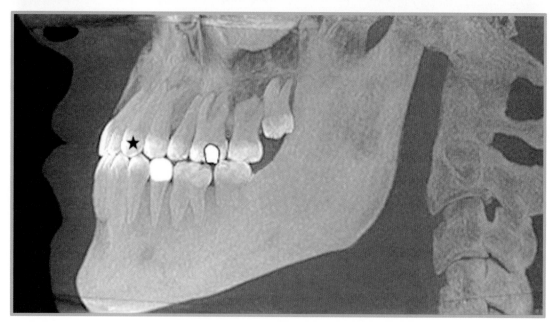

Spot eight differences between the sagittal images
Please see page 123 for solution

Puzzle 8

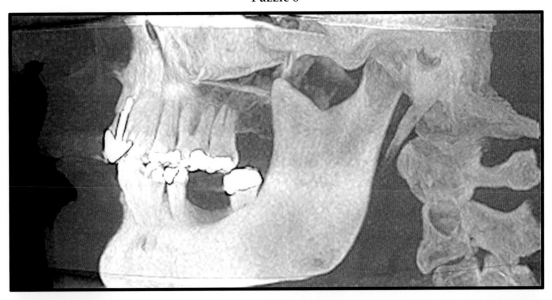

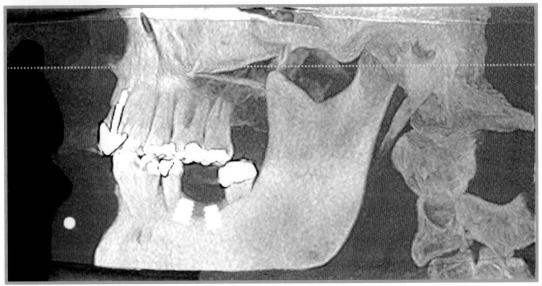

Spot nine differences between the sagittal images
Please see page 123 for solution

Puzzle 1 key

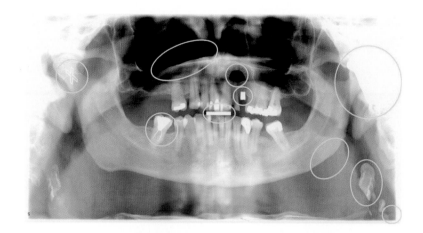

Puzzle 2 key

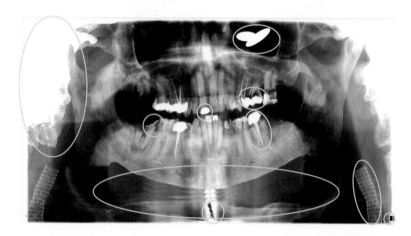

Puzzle 3 key

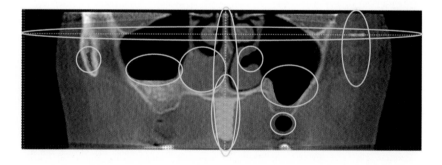

Puzzle 4 key

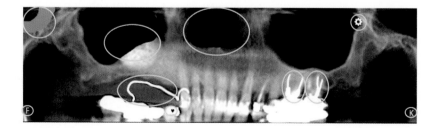

Puzzle 5 key

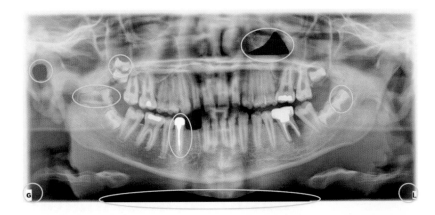

Puzzle 6 key

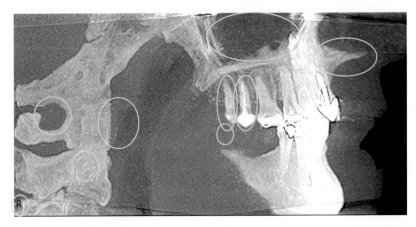

Puzzle 7 key

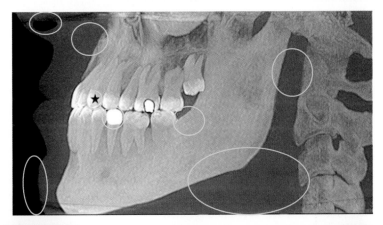

Puzzle 8 key

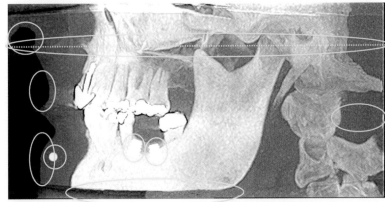

U

Radiographic Anatomy

Interpretation of abnormalities requires a thorough knowledge of normal anatomy. A comprehensive study of skull osteology cannot be covered within the scope of this textbook. Only the major landmarks commonly found on conventional dental x-ray images will be presented here.

Note: Natural skeletal variations between one patient and another can dramatically alter anatomic appearances. Variations in the operator's techniques, from positioning of the receptor to alignment of the PID, can dramatically distort or even obscure a landmark. Two-dimensional images of three-dimensional structures automatically result in object superimposition and panoramic imaging inherently produces *ghost images* which can easily lead to misinterpretation of normal anatomic landmarks.

1. DENTAL ANATOMY

Enamel (Fig. U1) is the most mineralized substance in the human body. Its 90% plus mineralization content is very effective at absorbing x radiation and as a result enamel typically appears as a thin radiopaque shell surrounding the crown of a tooth. It gradually tapers in thickness to a fine edge at the level of the cementum. It is noteworthy that the density and thickness of enamel is quite variable due to age, environment, congenital hypoplasia, etc.

Dentin (Fig. U1) is situated between the enamel and pulp and it is approximately two-thirds as mineralized as enamel. As a consequence, dentin will appear less radiopaque than enamel. It has a density comparable to bone. Generally the junction between enamel and dentin is distinguishable on x-ray images. However an x-ray image with poor contrast will make it difficult to differentiate dentin from enamel. Similar to enamel, dentin's density and thickness may be quite variable due to environmental and congenital factors.

Cementum is a thin calcified layer covering the root surface. It is approximately 50% mineralized. Differentiating cementum from dentin on an x-ray image is very difficult because the cementum layer is quite thin and its mineral content is similar to that of dentin. Hypercementosis, which is visible on x-ray images, is an alteration in the shape of a root. It occurs as a result of the deposition of variable amounts of secondary cementum.

Pulp (Fig. U1) is composed of vascularized and innervated soft tissue (i.e. connective tissue,

Fundamentals of Oral and Maxillofacial Radiology, First Edition. J. Sean Hubar.
© 2017 John Wiley & Sons, Inc. Published 2017 by John Wiley & Sons, Inc.
Companion website: www.wiley.com/go/hubar/radiology

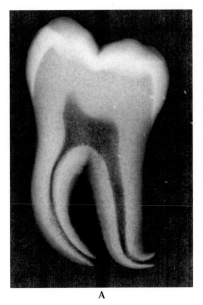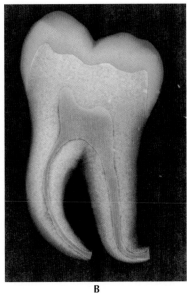

A   **B**

Fig. U1 Tooth structure. Red, enamel; grey, dentin; yellow, pulp chamber.

blood vessels, nerves). The term pulp is often used in lieu of pulp chamber or pulp canals. The pulp chamber and canals are hollowed cavities within the center of the tooth that extend from the coronal portion of the tooth to the apex of the root(s) which contains the pulpal tissue. A healthy pulp appears radiolucent in comparison with the dentin and enamel. The chamber and canals may become partially or fully calcified over time and as a result become radiopaque. Congenital maladies, natural aging and trauma contribute to dentin production, thus reducing the size of the pulp chamber. In addition, calcified *denticles* ☢ may form resulting in a reduction in the size of the pulp chamber.

Lamina dura (Fig. U2) is a thin radiopaque line that normally outlines the border of the entire tooth socket. It is merely a manifestation of x-ray beam absorption as the x rays pass through the socket wall and is not any more mineralized than normal trabecular bone. Many factors can alter the appearance or cause the disappearance of the lamina dura. It will typically appear very distinct and uniform if the horizontal

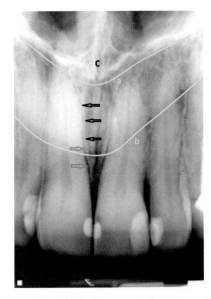

Fig. U2 Radiographic anatomy: a, outline of the soft tissue of the nose; it encompasses the uniformly faint radiopaque shadow superimposed over the roots of the maxillary central and lateral incisors; b, floor of the nasal fossa; c, anterior nasal spine (V-shaped radiopacity). The black arrows point to a thin radiopaque line which is the lamina dura. The red arrows point to a thin radiolucent line which is the periodontal ligament space.

angulation of the x-ray beam directly passes through the width (i.e. bucco-lingually) of the socket walls; whereas if the x-ray beam passes tangentially through the tooth socket, a smaller quantity of x rays will be absorbed and the lamina dura would be much less obvious or may not even be visible on an x-ray image. Additionally, if other anatomic structures are superimposed over the socket, these structures may disrupt the continuity of the lamina dura. Complete absence of the lamina dura may also be a sign of pathosis such as Paget's disease, fibrous dysplasia, osteopetrosis, osteosarcoma and hyperparathyroidism.

Periodontal ligament space (Fig. U2) is a thin radiolucent line located between the lamina dura and the root of a tooth on an x-ray image. It extends mesiodistally around the entire root, beginning and ending at the level of the alveolar crest. This radiolucent space contains the collagenous periodontal ligament which is not visible on x-ray images. The width of the periodontal ligament space (PDL space) can be quite variable even within the same individual. Similar to the variability in the thickness of the lamina dura, the PDL space may vary in width simply as a result the operator's intraoral technique. Modification of the horizontal angulation of the x-ray beam can alter the appearance of the PDL space. Occlusal biting forces or pathosis such as an osteosarcoma may also lead to abnormal widening of the PDL space.

Alveolar bone refers to the anatomic bone comprising the mandible and maxilla that surrounds and supports the dentition. Cortical bone (aka compact bone) is the dense shell of bone that forms the outer plates of both the maxilla and the mandible. Cortical bone appears as a thin radiopaque line of variable thickness. Trabecular bone (aka cancellous bone or spongy bone) is the bone that lies between the buccal and lingual cortical plates. Trabecular bone typically has a lace-like radiopaque appearance.

Alveolar crest is the superior aspect of the interproximal cortical plate of bone. It appears as a thin radiopaque line at the height of the alveolus spanning between adjacent teeth or along edentulous ridges. It may be horizontal or angled vertically. In a healthy dentition the alveolar crest runs parallel to and approximately one millimeter inferior to the cemento-enamel junction. Deviations from normal may be as a result of periodontal disease, etc. which may alter the height, angulation and thickness of the alveolar crest.

2. ANATOMIC LANDMARKS OF THE MAXILLARY REGION

Radiopaque landmarks

Anterior nasal spine (Fig. U2) is a midline bony projection located at the floor of the nasal cavity. It appears as a small *v-shaped* radiopacity. It is more easily observed on intraoral central incisor and lateral cephalometric projections. On panoramic images, the anterior nasal spine, the soft tissue of the nose and the oropharynx are frequently superimposed, which makes it difficult to discern.

Inverted "Y" or "X" (Fig. U3) produced by the intersection of the floor of the maxillary sinus and the nasal fossa. The radiolucent area to the right is the maxillary sinus and the radiolucent area to the left is the nasal fossa.

Nose (soft tissue) (Fig. U2) will often appear as a faint radiopaque shadow superimposed over the roots of the maxillary incisors on intraoral images. The *anterior nasal spine* ☢ will generally be superimposed over the soft tissue of the nose.

Nasal septum (Fig. U4) is the dividing wall composed of bone and cartilage that runs down the middle of the nasal fossa.

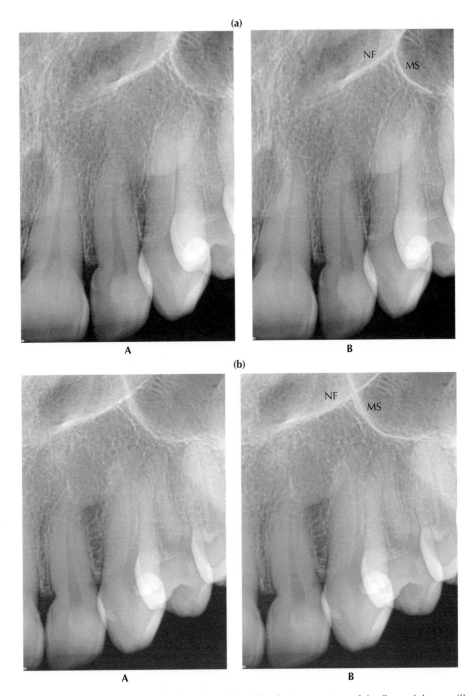

Fig. U3 **(a) Characteristic** inverted "Y" landmark produced by the intersection of the floor of the maxillary sinus and the nasal fossa. **(b)** Characteristic inverted "X" landmark produced by the intersection of the floor of the maxillary sinus (MS) and the nasal fossa (NF).

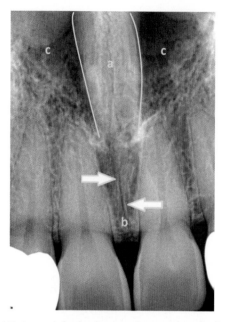

Fig. U4 Anatomic landmarks: a, nasal septum; b, mid-palatine suture appearing as a thin radiopaque line located between the maxillary central incisors; c, nasal fossa, which is the radiolucency extending superior to the incisors and bisected by the nasal septum.

Nasolabial folds (Fig. U5) are the bilateral folds of soft tissue extending from the lateral aspect of the nose to the corner of the mouth. Insertion of an intraoral receptor holder in the canine–premolar region will compress the soft tissue. Superimposition of this thick soft tissue over the teeth and bone will attenuate sufficient radiation so as to appear as a diffuse oblique radiopaque shadow extending posteriorly from the cuspid–premolar intraoral region. A sharp demarcation line will be observed at the anterior border of the nasolabial fold. The region anterior to the nasolabial fold will appear more radiolucent in comparison. In edentulous patients, this landmark can assist the operator in determining the right and left sides of the patient.

Pterygoid plates (medial and lateral) of the sphenoid bone (see Fig. M24) are best visualized on axial images. Intraoral images may or may not capture them because the plates are located posterior to the maxillary tuberosity. They will appear as uniform radiopacities without any

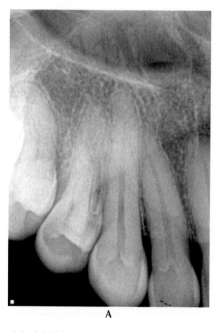
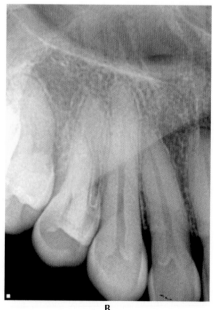

A   B

Fig. U5 Nasolabial fold (highlighted in B).

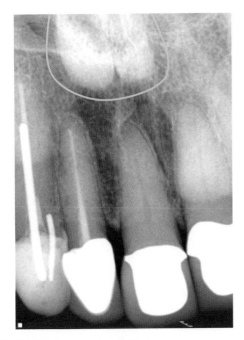

Fig. U6 Palatine torus (highlighted).

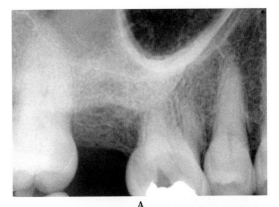

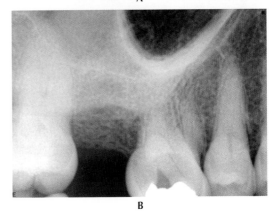

Fig. U7 Zygomatic arch (highlighted in B).

trabecular pattern. The hamular process extends off the medial pterygoid plate.

Palatine torus (pl. tori) (Fig. U6) is a bony protuberance located in the midline of the hard palate. It is quite a common phenomenon, occurring in approximately 20% of the population. A torus is typically less than 2 cm in diameter and may consist of several lobes of dense bone. A palatine torus usually appears as a dense radiopacity that may be partially super-imposed over the roots of posterior maxillary teeth. It often is misdiagnosed as the zygoma. Synonyms include torus palatinus and palatal torus.

Zygomatic arch (Fig. U7) is comprised of the zygoma and zygomatic process. The zygomatic process is actually an extension of the maxilla, temporal bone and frontal bone. In periapical images it appears as a *U-shaped* radiopacity in the first and second molar region. Generally, a portion of the maxillary sinus will be visible

behind it. Over- and underangulation of intraoral imaging techniques can dramatically vary the appearance of the zygomatic process. The zygoma appears as a uniform radiopacity continuing posteriorly from the zygomatic process. On intraoral images the inferior border of the zygoma will only be visible.

Radiolucent landmarks

Incisive foramen (Fig. U8) is the opening of the incisive canal located immediately behind the maxillary central incisors. The nasopalatine nerve and sphenopalatine artery exit through this foramen and supply the oral mucosa and hard palate. On periapical x-ray images, the

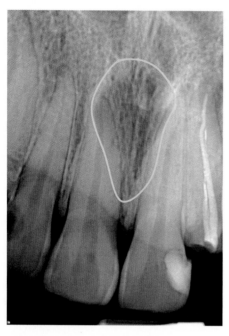

Fig. U8 Incisive foramen: appears as an elliptical radiolucency located between the roots of the central incisors (highlighted).

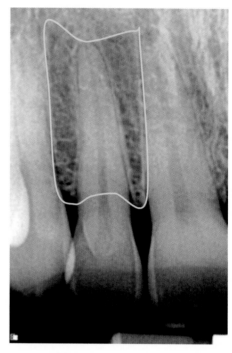

Fig. U9 Lateral fossa: appears as a diffuse radiolucency located around the root of a lateral incisor with an intact lamina dura (highlighted).

incisive foramen is located in the midline between the roots of the central incisors. Its appearance is quite variable due to normal anatomic variation and due to the operator's angulation of the x-ray beam. Typically it appears as a well-defined, round or elliptical radiolucency measuring up to 1 cm in diameter. Abnormal enlargement of the incisive foramen may be indicative of a nasopalatine cyst. Synonyms include nasopalatine foramen and anterior nasopalatine foramen.

Lateral fossa (Fig. U9) is a mild skeletal depression in the region of the maxillary lateral incisor. On a periapical image, the region may or may not appear slightly more radiolucent than the surrounding area. It should not be misdiagnosed as periapical pathology associated with a tooth. The lamina dura will typically be intact and clinically the patient will be asymptomatic. A synonym is incisive fossa.

Maxillary sinus (Figs U10 and U11) is the largest of the paranasal sinuses and is bilaterally located within the body of the maxilla. Each sinus is bounded by the zygoma and the body of the maxilla. The maxillary sinus extends anteriorly toward the canine. Posteriorly it may extend into the tuberosity region, often seen dipping interproximally between the roots of multiple teeth. Its size and shape is variable in appearance. Age and the loss of teeth contribute to increased *pneumatization* ☢ of a sinus, with the floor of the maxillary sinus possibly extending to the crest of the alveolar ridge. Within the maxillary sinus there is an ostium that connects the sinus to the middle concha of the nasal cavity. The maxillary sinuses typically appear as large radiolucencies outlined by a thin radiopaque border. Extraoral images such as panoramic and CBCT images project a full sinus view. However, with the limited field of view on periapical images, only the inferior aspect of the maxillary sinus will be visible. Superimposition of the floor of the nasal cavity over the maxillary sinus is often seen in periapical views of the canine. The intersection of the radiopaque borders of the sinus and the nasal cavity produces an inverted "Y" or "X" landmark. If the top of the image cuts off a segment of the intersecting lines, the intersecting lines will appear as a "Y"; if the intersecting lines are fully visible on the image, the result appears more like an "X". This landmark is useful to the operator to determine if a periorbital image belongs either to the right or left quadrant. This is particularly helpful for arranging x-ray images of edentulous patients. Actual interpretation of the intersecting inverted "Y" or "X" landmark is as follows: the oblique radiolucent region towards the anterior demarcates the nasal fossa, while the posterior radiolucency is the maxillary sinus.

The relationship of the maxillary sinus to the maxillary molars in particular is often misinterpreted. Two-dimensional images of teeth often appear to project the roots into the maxillary sinus when in fact the sinus is simply enveloping the roots and it is only superimposed over it. An analogy would be to poke your finger into a fully inflated balloon and then observe it from the side. Viewing the balloon from the side, it would give the illusion that your finger was actually inside the balloon, when in fact it was merely being enveloped by it. Advanced imaging techniques can accurately show their true relationship. An additional complicating effect that often is misdiagnosed as pathology where none exists also occurs when a sinus is

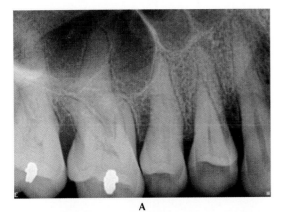

A

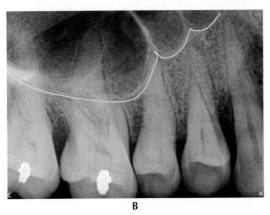

B

Fig. U10 Maxillary sinus (lower border highlighted in B).

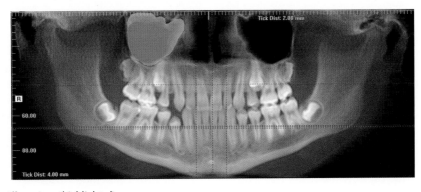

Fig. U11 Maxillary sinus (highlighted).

superimposed over a root. The effect is an illusionary widening of the PDL space around the apex. A normal radiolucent PDL space and the superimposed sinus together exaggerate the appearance of the PDL space. This may lead to misinterpretation as non-existent periapical pathology. Further clinical testing is necessary to rule out possible periapical pathology.

Within a healthy sinus there may appear to be thin radiolucent and radiopaque lines. The narrow radiolucent lines are called *nutrient canals* ☢, which carry the superior alveolar nerves and vessels, while the thin radiopaque lines are typically septa, which are simply undulating folds of cortical bone within the sinus. Neither should be considered pathogenic.

The maxillary sinuses are lined with a thin mucosal membrane. Inflammation of this mucosal lining can contribute to dental symptoms due to the close proximity of the apices of the molars to the inferior border of the sinus. Depending upon the degree of mucosal inflammation, the inferior portion of one or both maxillary sinuses may appear to be radiopaque. A thorough clinical examination of patients experiencing dental pain may reveal a healthy dentition with associated acute sinusitis.

Inadequate alveolar bone height for dental implant placement often calls for a *sinus lift* ☢ procedure with bone augmentation using autogenous or alloplastic materials (see Fig. Y14). In post-sinus lift surgery, the inferior aspect of the grafted sinus material typically appears as a uniformly dense, irregular or dome-shaped radiopacity. This radiopacity must not be confused with a mucocele within the sinus, which is a simply a build-up of fluids. On rare occasions, there may be *aplasia* ☢ of the maxillary sinus or complete opacification of the sinuses.

Mid-palatine suture (Fig. U4) is the line of union between the horizontal plates of the palatine bone. It typically appears as a thin radiolucent line extending from the incisive canal posteriorly. On a periapical x-ray image of the central incisors, it will often appear to extend from the alveolar crest superiorly up to the anterior nasal septum. However, its visibility on an x-ray image is particularly dependent upon the horizontal angulation of the x-ray beam. Directing the x-ray beam diagonally through the thin mid-palatine suture may obscure it because the suture line will now be superimposed with the denser surrounding palatal bone. Synonyms include intermaxillary suture, median palatine suture and palatomaxillary suture.

Nasal fossa (Fig. U4) is the large midline air space that extends anteroposteriorly from the nares into the nasopharynx. It is divided into two compartments by the nasal septum. It is bounded superiorly by the cribiform plate of the ethmoid bone and inferiorly by the processes of the maxilla and the horizontal portion of the palatine bone. The lateral walls of the fossa each have three *conchae* ☢ (synonym: turbinates): the superior, middle and inferior conchae. Anterior periapical x-ray images often will capture a portion of the inferior aspect of the nasal fossa. Its presence or absence will vary greatly depending on the extent of the vertical angulation of the x-ray beam. In the central incisor region, the inferior border of the fossa will typically appear as a V-shaped radiopaque line located well above the apices of the teeth. The nasal septum appears in the midline as a radiopaque line rising vertically from the inferior border of the nasal fossa. The adjoining air space of the nasal cavity will appear radiolucent and it will be bisected by the nasal septum. The maxillary cuspid periapical view often contains the floor of the nasal fossa intersecting with the floor of the maxillary sinus, forming an inverted "Y" or "X" configuration (Fig. U3). The nasal conchae will be more visible on extraoral imaging of the nasal fossa. The conchae will appear as elongated radiopacities extending the length of the nasal cavity in sagittal views, while in cross-sectional views the conchae appear more semicircular, like the musical symbol "bass clef." Synonyms include nasal cavity and nasal antrum.

3. ANATOMIC LANDMARKS OF THE MANDIBULAR REGION

Radiopaque landmarks

Coronoid process (Fig. U12) is the thin, triangular-shaped process of the anterosuperior aspect of the ramus. Its triangular shape resembles the dorsal fin of a shark. This mandibular landmark is typically observed in extraoral images. However, it may also appear in maxillary molar periapical images. This can occur because the mandible must swing open to accommodate the intraoral receptor holder. In so doing, the coronoid process rotates anteroinferiorly and often becomes superimposed over the maxillary molar tuberosity region. The coronoid process appears as a homogeneous triangular radiopacity.

Genial tubercles (Fig. U13) are small bony projections in the midline on the lingual aspect of the mandible. The genioglossus and geniohyoid muscles attach at these points. They are quite variable in appearance. On mandibular incisor periapical images, the genial tubercles may appear as a donut-shaped radiopacity several millimeters in diameter with a pin-point radiolucent center (i.e. *lingual foramen* ☢). On axial CBCT images and mandibular occlusal images, the genial tubercles will typically appear as small projections emanating from the lingual cortical plate. A synonym is mental spine.

Inferior border (i.e. cortical plate) of the mandible (Fig. U14) appears as a uniformly dense radiopaque band. On periapical x-ray images, it should not be confused with either the external or the internal oblique ridges. Generally, the inferior border of the mandible is not observed on periapical images unless there was excessive negative vertical angulation of the x-ray beam.

Lip line (Fig. U15) is the result of the soft tissue of the lip attenuating enough radiation to be visible on a periapical image of the anterior teeth. The lip line is recognized by a uniform change in density horizontally across the coronal portions of teeth. The more radiolucent portion of the crown is superior to the lip line.

Mental ridge (Fig. U16) is a dense elevation on the anterolateral aspect of the body of the mandible. On anterior periapical images, it appears

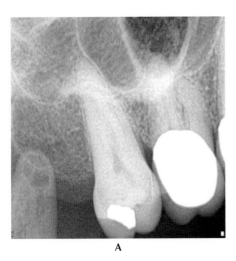
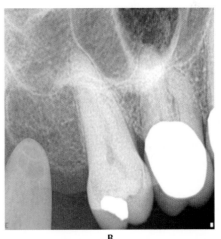

A   B

Fig. U12 Coronoid process: appears as a triangular-shaped radiopacity located in a maxillary molar periapical (highlighted in B).

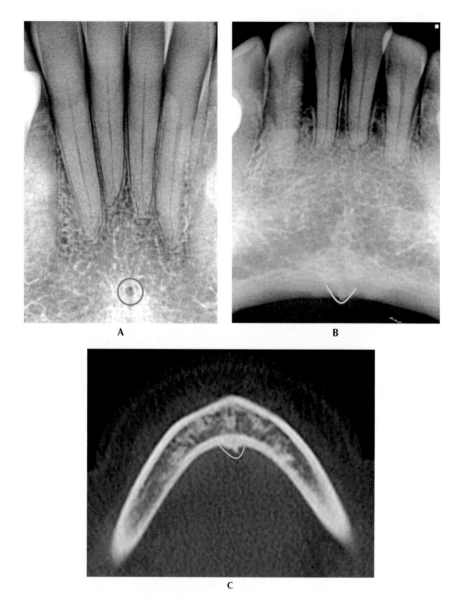

Fig. U13 Genial tubercles. A. The genial tubercles appear as a radiopaque circle. The small radiolucency within the genial tubercles is the lingual foramen. B. Increased vertical angulation of the PID results in the genial tubercles appearing as a spiny process. C. The genial tubercles appear as a spiny process in an axial view.

as a thin radiopaque line extending posteriorly from the midline (i.e. bilaterally). It usually is located inferior to the teeth, but if excessive negative vertical angulation of the x-ray beam occurs, the mental ridge will be superimposed over the mandibular anterior teeth. A synonym is mental process.

External oblique ridge (Fig. U17) is the bony protuberance that extends off the anterolateral

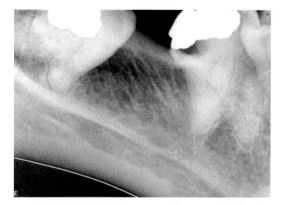

Fig. U14 Inferior border of the mandible (highlighted).

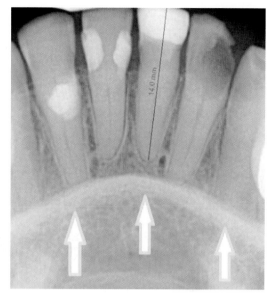

Fig. U16 Mental ridge (arrows).

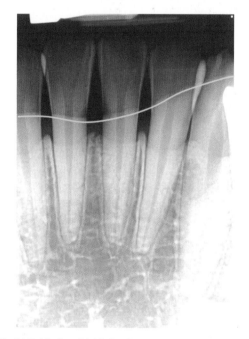

Fig. U15 Lip line (highlighted).

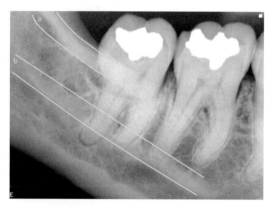

Fig. U17 External oblique ridge (a) and internal oblique ridge (b) (synonym: mylohyoid ridge).

border of the ramus and runs diagonally towards the area of the first molar. It serves as an attachment site of the buccinator muscle. The external oblique ridge typically appears to run parallel and superior to the internal oblique ridge. It appears as a thin oblique radiopaque line that gradually disappears as it extends from the ramus to approximately the location of the first molar.

Internal oblique ridge (Fig. U17) is the bony protuberance located on the lingual surface of mandible extending diagonally downward from the ramus and ending anteriorly near the apices of the premolars. Its function is to serve as an attachment site for the mylohyoid muscle of the floor of the mouth. The appearance of the internal oblique ridge can be quite variable. On periapical images, it may appear to be a well-defined, thin radiopaque line located inferior to the external oblique ridge. It runs obliquely at the level of the apices of the molars and premolars from the ramus. In some individuals, the internal oblique ridge may be quite diffuse and indistinguishable from the surrounding alveolar bone. A synonym is mylohyoid ridge.

Mandibular torus (pl. tori) (Fig. U18) is a bony protuberance located on the lingual side of the mandible, typically found bilaterally in the cuspid and premolar region. It occurs less commonly than the palatine torus (i.e. in approximately 8% versus 20% of the population). A mandibular torus typically appears as a rounded uniform radiopacity. The size of a torus is quite variable. Occasionally, bilateral tori together may fill the floor of the mouth. Placement of solid-state receptors for intraoral images may be physically impossible due to space limitation. PSP plates, which are comparatively thinner and more flexible, may be an alternative if available. Otherwise extraoral imaging (e.g. panoramic image) may be the only practical method to image the teeth. A synonym is torus mandibularis.

Radiolucent landmarks

Lingual foramen (Fig. U13) is a small foramen that the lingual artery passes through. It is situated on the lingual side in the midline of the mandible. Typically on periapical images of the mandibular anterior region, the lingual foramen will appear as a pinpoint radiolucency surrounded by the radiopaque genial tubercles. The small size and location of the lingual foramen often make it difficult to visualize on x-ray images.

Mandibular canal (Figs U19 and U20) extends from the mandibular foramen to the mental foramen through the ramus and body of the mandible. The inferior alveolar nerve and artery travel within this canal. An extension of the mandibular canal can sometimes be seen

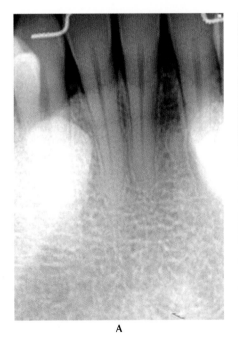
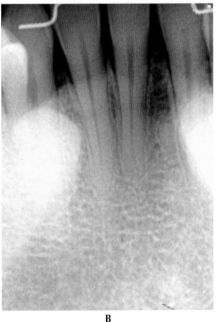

A   B

Fig. U18 Bilateral mandibular tori (highlighted in B).

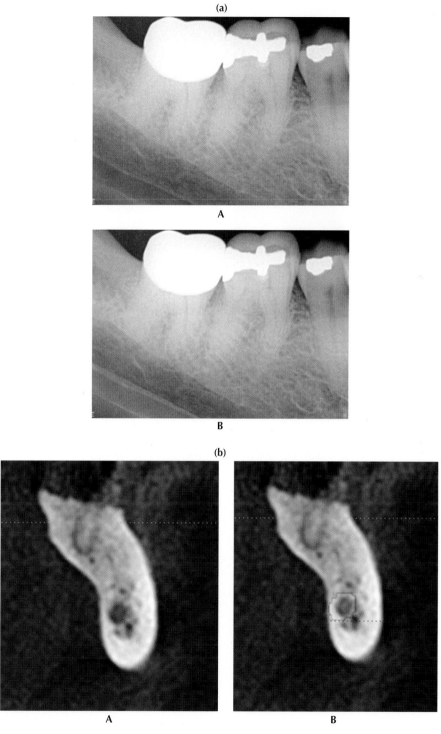

Fig. U19 (a) Mandibular canal (highlighted in B): conventional x-ray image. **(b)** Mandibular canal (highlighted in B): CBCT coronal view.

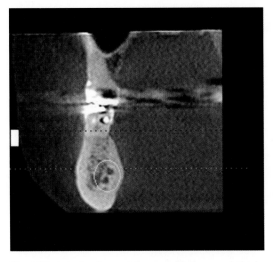

Fig. U20 Anterior loop of the mandibular canal (highlighted): CBCT coronal view.

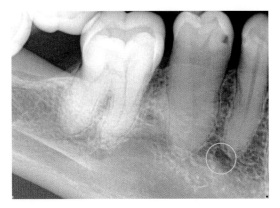

Fig. U21 Mental foramen (highlighted).

continuing anteriorly beyond the mental foramen. This is referred to as the *anterior loop of the mandibular canal* ☢☢. The mandibular canal typically traverses the body of the mandible inferior to the apices of the molars and premolars. Excessive negative vertical angulation of the x-ray beam may superimpose the mandibular canal over the apices of some teeth in periapical images. The mandibular canal typically is a uniform radiolucent channel bordered with thin parallel radiopaque lines. At times, the density of the mandibular canal may be indistinguishable from the surrounding bone. This will be a particular concern when treatment planning mandibular implants. A dental implant that impinges on the mandibular canal may lead to long-term *paresthesia* ☢☢. On occasion, a second mandibular canal may be observed running parallel to the primary canal. The second canal contains smaller branches of the inferior alveolar nerve. It is referred to as a *bifid canal* ☢☢ and is more frequently visualized on extraoral images such as panoramic or CBCT views. A bifid canal may result in the inability of the practitioner to fully anaesthetize a patient while performing mandibular dental procedures. A synonym is the inferior alveolar canal.

Mental foramen (Fig. U21) is the anterior opening of the mandibular canal allowing a branch of the inferior alveolar nerve and artery to exit into the facial soft tissue. It is bilaterally located on the buccal surface of the mandible in the premolar region. The mental foramen typically appears as a single round radiolucency in close proximity to the apices of the second premolar. However, its position on periapical images is very technique sensitive, being dependent upon both the vertical and horizontal angulation of the x-ray beam. Occasionally the image of the mental foramen may be superimposed over the apex of one of the premolars. This could easily be misdiagnosed as periapical pathology. Careful examination of the image should reveal an intact lamina dura of a vital tooth beneath the mental foramen. To rule out pulpal pathology, the operator may expose an additional x-ray image using a modified vertical or horizontal angulation of the x-ray beam. If the apical radiolucency drifts off of the tooth, this would indicate that it was most likely the mental foramen. However, if the radiolucency remains attached to the apex after a significant modification of the x-ray beam angulation, it would seem to indicate that some periapical pathology is present and further evaluation is prudent. Clinical testing for pulp vitality should be done.

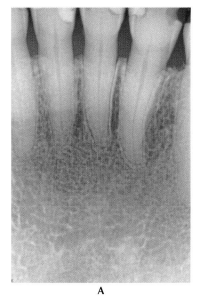 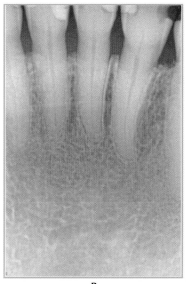

A   B

Fig. U22 Mental fossa (highlighted in B).

Mental fossa (Fig. U22) is an anatomic depression in the midline of the mandible superior to the mental ridge. The definition of a depression presumes less bone thickness. Prominence or lack thereof of a patient's mental protuberance will result in visibility or invisibility of the mental fossa on an x-ray image. If there is sufficient difference in bony thickness between the mental fossa and the surrounding bone, the fossa will appear comparatively more radiolucent. If there is insufficient difference in bone thickness, the mental fossa will not be discernable.

Nutrient canals (Fig. U23) are naturally occurring channels within bone that carry accessory blood vessels. They appear as thin radiolucent lines occurring in either the mandible or the maxilla. However, they are most commonly seen running vertically in the inter-radicular spaces between mandibular anterior teeth. If a nutrient canal is orientated bucco-lingually in the image, it will appear as a small round radiolucency.

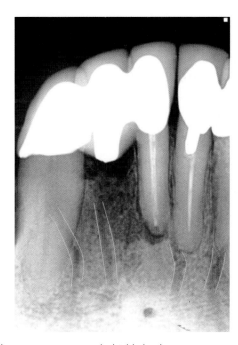

Fig. U23 Nutrient canals (highlighted).

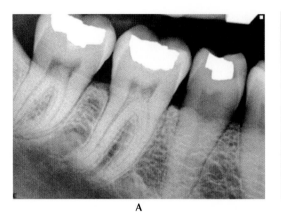 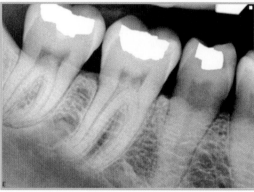

A   B

Fig. U24 Submandibular gland fossa (highlighted in B).

Submandibular gland fossa (Fig. U24) is a depression on the lingual side of the mandible body in the molar region and inferior to the internal oblique ridge (aka mylohyoid ridge). The submandibular salivary gland is situated in the fossa. Unlike the mental fossa, where there may not be an adequate difference in thickness of surrounding bone to distinguish it, the submandibular gland fossa usually is significantly thinner. Consequently the submandibular gland fossa is generally discernible on an x-ray image. The clinician must be cognizant that the radiolucent region associated with the submandibular gland is not osseous pathology.

V

Dental Caries

Dental caries (aka dental cavity or tooth decay) is a disease process of the calcified tissues of teeth. Contributing etiologic factors include diet, oral hygiene, composition of tooth structure and saliva. Caries may be single or multiple in number and may occur in both the deciduous and permanent dentitions. There is no age, sex or racial predilection. The size of the lesion is variable, ranging from under a millimeter to total destruction of a tooth. Clinically, the appearance varies from a white chalky area on the enamel to a large hollowed-out, darkly stained cavity. Depending upon the location and stage of caries development, its appearance is extremely variable. It is important to state outright that both an x-ray examination and a clinical oral examination are necessary to properly diagnose dental caries.

Limitations to visualizing caries on x-ray images

Decalcification levels

X-ray receptors require approximately a 40% decalcification of tooth structure prior to being able to detect a change. Consequently, early stages of caries development will not be visible on x-ray images. Since minute levels of decalcification are not detected with an x-ray receptor, lesions will automatically appear smaller on an x-ray image than they are clinically. This becomes a concern when a caries is encroaching upon the pulp chamber. A thin dentin separation between the active caries and the pulp may be visible on the x-ray image, but, in actuality, the caries may have already penetrated into the pulp.

Incorrect angulation of equipment

Caries detection may be impossible to visualize if incorrect angulation of the PID occurs. Incorrect horizontal angulation will superimpose adjacent proximal contacts over one another, which will likely obscure *incipient caries* ☢. Similarly, excessive vertical angulation will project caries through additional tooth structure and possibly behind radiopaque restorations making some caries undetectable on the x-ray image (Fig. V1).

Anatomy

Physical and anatomic factors may prevent an operator from positioning the x-ray receptor anteriorly enough to capture the contact between

Fundamentals of Oral and Maxillofacial Radiology, First Edition. J. Sean Hubar.
© 2017 John Wiley & Sons, Inc. Published 2017 by John Wiley & Sons, Inc.
Companion website: www.wiley.com/go/hubar/radiology

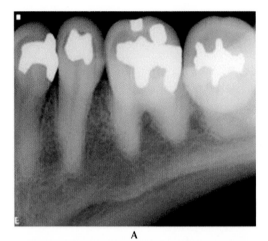

A

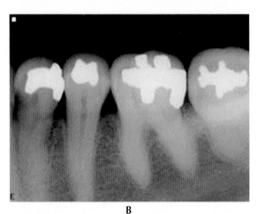

B

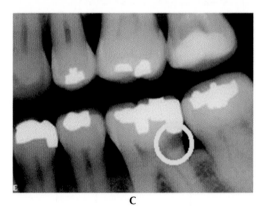

C

Fig. V1 Effect of overangulation. A. The caries is undetected on no. 19 because of excessive vertical angulation of the PID. B. The caries still undetected on no. 19 with reduced vertical angulation. C. Zero vertical angulation reveals a large carious lesion previously hidden on no. 19.

the first premolar and cuspid. This may be the result of the patient's mandibular and maxillary arch anatomy, which can restrict the placement of the receptor. Another impediment may be the sheer size and rigidity of the solid-state image receptor. PSP plates, if available, would facilitate placement in this situation. Similarly, tooth crowding and tooth rotation may prevent the operator from positioning the PID properly to open the contacts for caries detection.

Artifacts

Artifacts such as cervical burnout and the Mach band effect can lead to the misdiagnosis of x-ray images. The *Mach band effect* ☢ is an illusionary radiolucent line sometimes seen along the borders of dentin and enamel or along the border of a radiopaque restoration and normal tooth structure. *Cervical burnout* is an illusionary radiolucency along the neck of the tooth caused by differential x-ray absorption. More x rays penetrate through the cervical region, giving that area a more radiolucent appearance compared to the crown or the root. Cervical burnout can form a radiolucent band extending mesiodistally across the entire tooth or it can be localized to smaller areas in the mesial and/or distal surfaces along the neck of the tooth. None of these artifacts should be misdiagnosed as dental caries. Conversely, root surface caries should not be misdiagnosed as cervical burnout.

Viewing conditions

Viewing conditions can affect the quality of the x-ray images. A high resolution x-ray image that is viewed on a mediocre computer monitor will diminish the overall image quality. In addition, the viewing room itself, if brightly lit, can diminish the clinician's ability to visualize fine details and may lead to missed diagnoses.

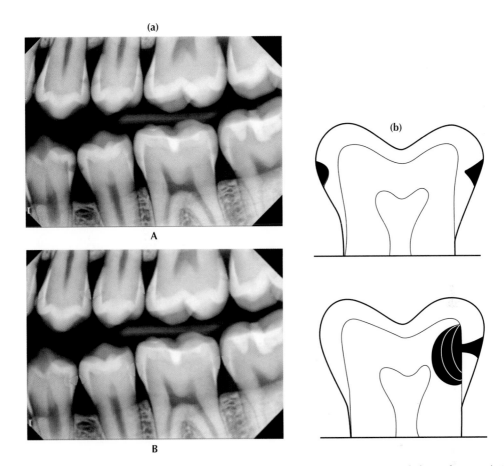

Fig. V2 (a) Interproximal caries (highlighted in B). (Source: Courtesy of Adam Chen, XDR Radiology.) **(b)** An early inter-proximal caries forms a triangle in the enamel with the broad base of the triangle located at the outer surface and the apex directed towards the dento-enamel junction. Progression of caries in the dentin similarly forms a broad base at the dento-enamel junction with the apex pointing toward the pulp.

Note: Caries detection can be enhanced by selecting lower kilovoltage settings for intra-oral imaging. A lower kilovoltage output produces an image with a more black–white contrast and fewer shades of gray.

shaped radiolucencies. Definitive diagnosis of buccal and lingual caries can be achieved by conducting a clinical exam. Clinically this type of caries is often associated with enamel pits and fissures.

Classification of caries

Buccal and lingual caries

Buccal and lingual caries typically appear as round or oval-shaped radiolucencies with well-defined margins, while cemental caries generally appear as well-defined saucer-

Interproximal caries

An interproximal caries is first evident as a triangular radiolucency in the enamel with the base of the triangle along the outer surface of the tooth and the apex of the triangle pointing toward the dentin (Fig. V2b). At the dentin–enamel junction, a second similarly orientated

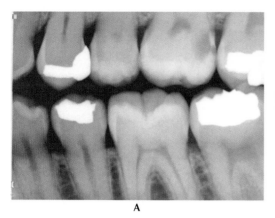
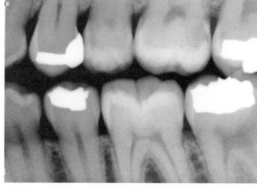

A   B

Fig. V3 Interproximal caries (highlighted in B).

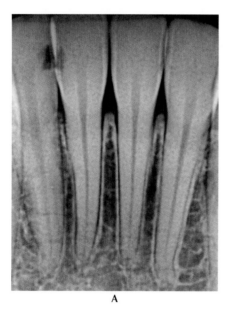
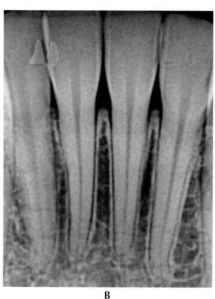

A   B

Fig. V4 Interproximal caries (highlighted in B).

radiolucent triangle will form (i.e. the base located at the dentin–enamel junction and the apex pointing toward the pulp chamber). As it progressively enlarges and begins to encroach upon the pulp chamber, it will lose its triangular shape and become irregular in outline (Figs V3 and V4). Bitewing images are ideally suited for diagnosing interproximal caries.

Occlusal caries

An occlusal caries classically forms a triangular-shaped radiolucency in the enamel with the triangle's apex at the outer surface of the crown and its base located along the dentin–enamel junction. As it progresses into the dentin, it forms an additional opposing triangle with the base also located at the dentin–enamel junction. Identical

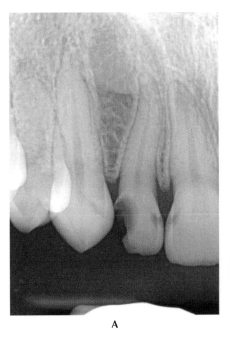 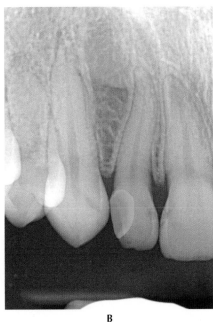

A B

Fig. V5 Interproximal caries (highlighted in B).

to interproximal caries, the triangle's apex points inward towards the pulp chamber (Fig. V6b). These caries will continue to spread laterally in the dentin, undermining the enamel and will transform it into a large, irregular-shaped radiolucent lesion (Figs V6 and V7). At some juncture the undermined enamel will break away, clinically revealing a large open cavity (Fig. V8).

Radiation caries

Medical radiotherapy for the treatment of head and neck cancer can result in loss of function of the salivary glands causing dry mouth (aka xerostomia). Reduced salivary flow increases the risk for dental caries. The phenomenon is referred to as *radiation caries*, where the caries are indirectly the result of the radiation treatment and not directly due to the radiation itself. The result can be rampant caries with total destruction of the coronal portions of the teeth. There are limited options to protect the teeth in patients undergoing therapeutic radiation for

head and neck cancer. Teeth will require meticulous oral hygiene care and may be treated with topical fluorides and artificial saliva.

Recurrent caries

Recurrent caries (aka secondary caries) refers to active caries associated with an existing dental restoration. A radiolucency particularly associated with the proximal surface of an existing restoration may be a new carious lesion that requires retreatment. However, not all radiolucencies associated with restorations are active caries. The radiolucency can possibly be a liner that was intentionally placed at the time underneath the restoration. If the depth of the caries was close to the pulp chamber, the restoring clinician may have intentionally left some caries behind and lined it with the medicament. Without an x-ray image and clinical history of an existing restoration, a new dentist cannot determine if the radiolucency associated with the restoration is an active caries. An active caries requires proper treatment.

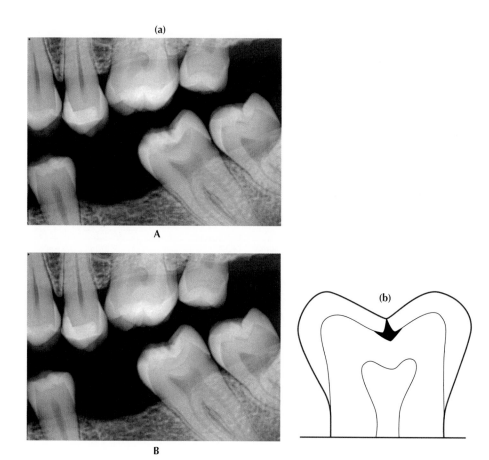

Fig. V6 (a) Occlusal caries (highlighted in B). (Source: Courtesy of Adam Chen, XDR Radiology.) **(b)** An early occlusal caries forms a triangle in the enamel with the apex of the triangle located at the outer surface and the broad base directed towards the dento-enamel junction. Progression of the caries in the dentin forms a broad base at the dento-enamel junction with the apex pointing toward the pulp.

Root surface caries

Root surface caries (synonym: cemental caries) is associated with gingival recession and crestal alveolar bone loss. It affects the dentin and cementum together and it should be evident clinically. X-ray images should not even be required for its diagnosis. When x-ray images are available, a root surface caries has a diffuse periphery and may have a saucer shape (Fig. V9). Root surface caries should not be misdiagnosed as cervical burnout (Fig. V10).

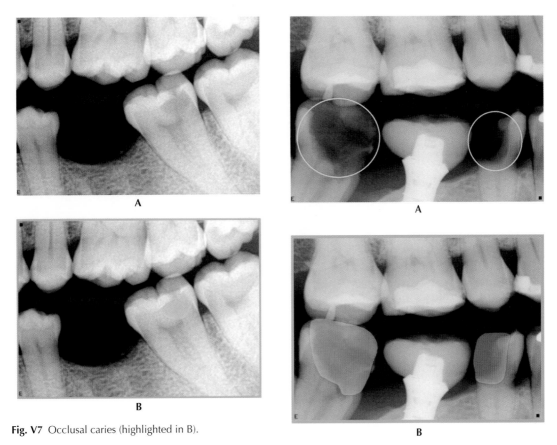

Fig. V7 Occlusal caries (highlighted in B).

Fig. V8 Severe caries (highlighted in B).

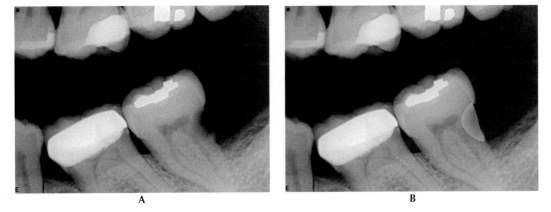

Fig. V9 Root caries (highlighted in B).

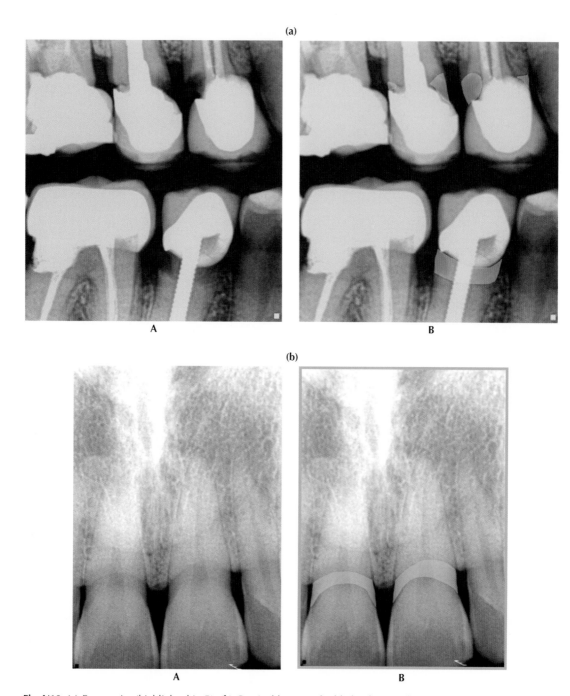

Fig. V10 (a) Root caries (highlighted in B). **(b)** Cervical burnout (highlighted in B). This must not be misdiagnosed as root caries.

W | **Dental Anomalies**

Number

Anodontia (Fig. W1)

Anodontia is the congenital absence of all deciduous and/or permanent teeth. It is a rare condition, often associated with other disorders such as *ectodermal dysplasia* ☢, progeria or Down's syndrome. Females are more often affected, but there is no racial predilection. Synonyms include *hypodontia* and *agenesis of teeth*.

Oligodontia (Fig. W2)

Oligodontia is the congenital absence of one or more deciduous or permanent teeth. The maxillary and mandibular third molars, the maxillary lateral incisors and the mandibular second premolars are the most frequent congenitally absent permanent teeth, while the maxillary and mandibular lateral incisors and the mandibular cuspids are the most frequently absent deciduous teeth. Oligodontia is often associated with other disorders such as anhidrotic ectodermal dysplasia, chondro-ectodermal dysplasia, oro-digitofacial dysostosis and Down's syndrome. Synonyms include *partial anodontia* and *hypodontia*.

Supernumerary tooth (Fig. W3)

Supernumerary tooth/teeth refer to the presence of one or more teeth in excess of the normal complement. Although supernumerary teeth are more prevalent in males, there is no age or racial predilection. They are often small rudimentary teeth, single or multiple and may be found in any of the tooth-bearing areas of the jaws. However, the area between the maxillary central incisors, the area distal to the third molars and the mandibular bicuspid regions are the most common sites for supernumerary teeth. Clinically, the patient may present with malocclusion. Synonyms include *mesiodens*, *peridens*, *hyperdontia* and *supplemental teeth*.

Size

Macrodontia (Fig. W4)

Macrodontia is a term used to describe one or more deciduous or permanent teeth that appear normal in every respect, except for their large size. They may be found in any of the tooth-bearing areas of the maxilla and mandible and in individuals of all ages. They are often associated with giantism and unilateral

Fundamentals of Oral and Maxillofacial Radiology, First Edition. J. Sean Hubar.
© 2017 John Wiley & Sons, Inc. Published 2017 by John Wiley & Sons, Inc.
Companion website: www.wiley.com/go/hubar/radiology

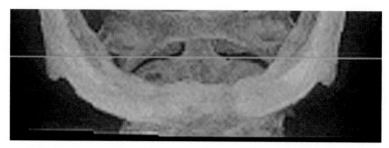

Fig. W1 Anodontia.

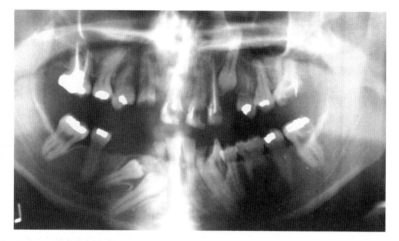

Fig. W2 Oligodontia.

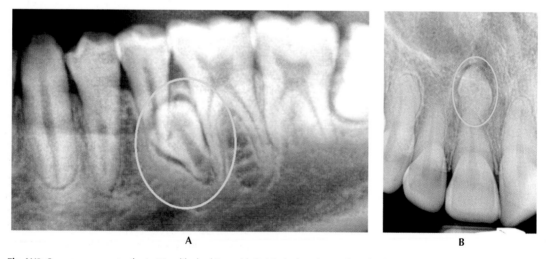

Fig. W3 Supernumerary teeth. A. Mandibular bicuspid. B. Mesiodens (e.g. microdont).

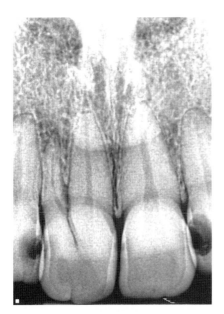

Fig. W4 Macrodontia (e.g. fusion).

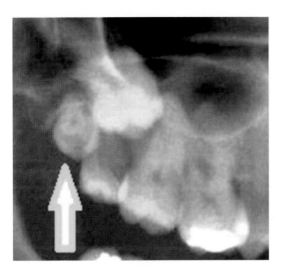

Fig. W5 Microdontia.

hypertrophy of the face. Synonyms include *megalodontia* and *megadontia*.

Microdontia (Fig. W5)

Microdontia is a term used to describe one or more deciduous or permanent teeth that appear normal in every respect, except for their small size. They can be found in any of the tooth-bearing areas of the jaws and in individuals of all ages. Particularly affected are the maxillary lateral incisors and maxillary third molars in the permanent dentitions. In addition, they are often associated with osteogenesis imperfecta and Down's syndrome. Synonyms include *dwarf teeth* and *peg laterals*.

Shape

Concrescence (Fig. W6)

Concrescence is the union of either two deciduous or two permanent teeth by cementum alone. There are occasional reports of cases in which

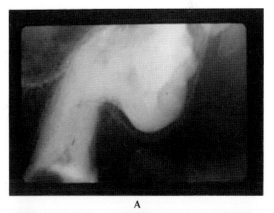

A

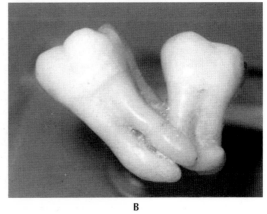

B

Fig. W6 Concrescence. (Source: Courtesy of Dr. K. Thunthy.)

three teeth are joined together by cementum. The maxillary molars are the most frequently affected teeth and, although the etiology is unknown, there is often a history of trauma to the area or severe crowding of the dentition. There is no age, sex or racial predilection. Concrescence appears as two fused teeth having amorphous roots, and often one of those teeth is unerupted. It is notable that the diagnosis of concrescence using x-ray images alone is often impossible.

Dens invaginatus (Fig. W7)

Dens invaginatus is a developmental anomaly believed to arise from an invagination in the surface of the crown of a permanent tooth before calcification has occurred. The maxillary lateral incisors are most frequently affected. Dens invaginatus often appears as a "pear-shaped"

radiolucent invagination lined with a thin layer of enamel and dentin that projects into the pulp. There is no age, sex or racial predilection. Clinically, the patient often presents with pain and/or a periapical abscess. Synonyms include *dens in dente*, *dilated composite odontome* and *gestant odontome*.

Denticle (Fig. W8)

A *denticle* is a round or oval-shaped calcified body within a pulp chamber of either a permanent or deciduous tooth. It appears as a uniform, dense, radiopaque mass with well-defined borders. Its size can range from 1 mm in diameter to total obliteration of the pulp chamber. Clinically, there is no age or racial predilection and it is usually asymptomatic. Synonyms include *pulp stone*, *pulp nodule* and *endolith*.

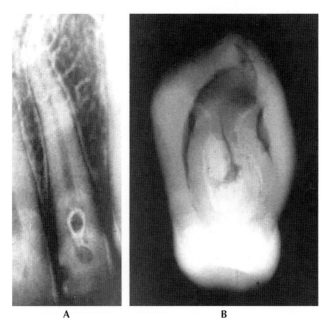

A B

Fig. W7 Dens invaginatus. A. Lateral incisor. B. Holar. (Source: Courtesy of Dr. K. Thunthy.)

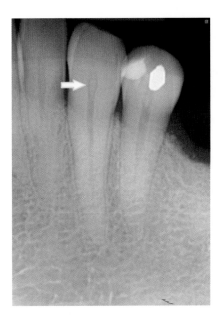

Fig. W8 Denticle.

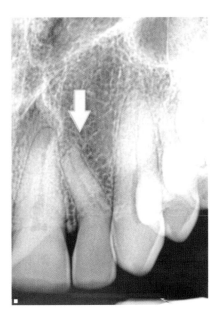

Fig. W10 Dilaceration.

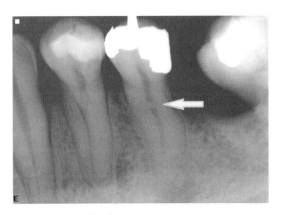

Fig. W9 Dentinal bridge.

Dentinal bridge (Fig. W9)

A *dentinal bridge* is a partial obliteration of a pulp chamber of either a deciduous or permanent tooth. Typically only a single tooth is involved. There is no racial or sexual predilection and it may be diagnosed in any age group. It appears as a narrow radiopaque band spanning horizontally across the pulp chamber. The thickness of the band is variable, ranging from one to several millimeters in width. Clinically, the affected tooth is asymptomatic.

Dilaceration (Fig. W10)

Dilaceration refers to an abnormal distortion either in the root of a tooth or at a junction of the crown and root of a tooth. The etiology is believed to be trauma during tooth development. It may occur in either the permanent or the deciduous dentition, but it is more frequently found in permanent teeth. There is no sexual or racial predilection and it may be diagnosed in any age group. The tooth appears normal except that its shape is bent or twisted. Clinically, dilaceration is asymptomatic.

Enamel pearl (Fig. W11)

An *enamel pearl* is a small hemispherical mass of enamel attached to the surface of a permanent tooth. Typically, it is a single globular mass found at the cemento-enamel

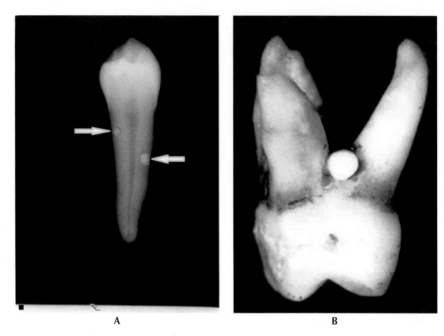

Fig. W11 Enamel pearl. (B. Source: Courtesy of Dr. K. Thunthy.)

junction in or near the bifurcation or trifurcation of the roots of the posterior teeth, particularly the maxillary first molar. The average size of the enamel pearl varies from 1 to 5 mm. There is no sex predilection. The enamel pearl appears as a well-defined, round or ovoid, dense radiopacity with or without a normal lamina dura and a periodontal ligament-like space present. Clinically, it is usually asymptomatic. Synonyms include *enameloma*, *enamel nodule* and *enamel drop*.

Fusion (Fig. W4)

Fusion is either the partial or complete union of two deciduous or permanent teeth. Although its etiology is uncertain, fusion is believed to be hereditary. The mandibular and maxillary anterior deciduous teeth are most frequently affected, but there is no age, sex or racial predilection. In addition to affecting two normal teeth, fusion may occur between a supernumerary tooth and a normal tooth. It resembles a macrodont tooth, except that fused teeth often have two pulp chambers. Clinically, there is at least one tooth missing from the normal complement of teeth. A synonym is *synodontia*.

Gemination (Fig. W12)

Gemination is a developmental anomaly in which a single tooth bud attempts to divide by invagination, resulting in incomplete formation of two teeth. There is a predilection for the maxillary and mandibular anterior deciduous dentition, with rare reports of occurrence in the permanent dentition. Consequently, geminated teeth may be found in any age group but occur more frequently in children under 12 years of age; there is no sexual or racial predilection. The teeth appear normal except for atypically large crowns. Unlike fusion, there is often a full complement of teeth present.

Hutchinson's incisor (Fig. W13)

A *Hutchinson's incisor* refers to a characteristic screwdriver shape and/or notching of the incisal edges of permanent maxillary and mandibular incisors. Hutchinson's incisors appear normal except for an irregular border of the incisal edges. Clinically, there is no racial or sexual predilection, and it is rarely diagnosed in children below 6 years of age. Hutchinson's incisors are associated with congenital syphilis, interstitial keratitis and deafness. A synonym is *screwdriver tooth*.

Hypercementosis (Fig. W14)

Hypercementosis is an alteration in the shape of a root of a permanent tooth as a result of the deposition of excessive amounts of secondary cementum. It is often described as "clubshaped." Regardless of the shape of the altered root, it always maintains the normal width of

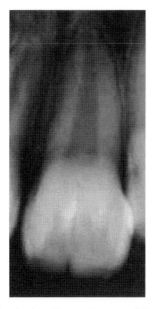

Fig. W12 Gemination. (Source: Courtesy of Dr. K. Thunthy.)

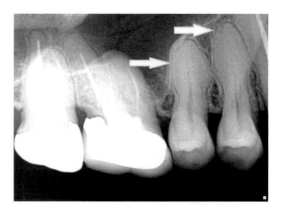

Fig. W14 Hypercementosis.

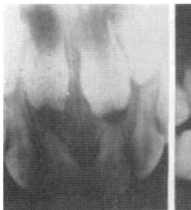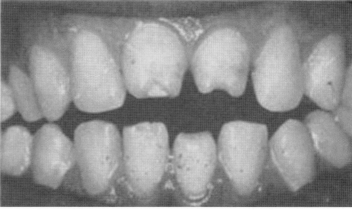

Fig. W13 Hutchinson's incisors. (Source: Courtesy of T. Putkonen.)

the lamina dura and periodontal membrane around it. Secondary cementum may form over the entire root surface or focally in one area. Because cementum is less radiopaque than dentin, the border between the two is distinguishable. Hypercementosis primarily affects the premolar and molar teeth. There is a higher incidence of occurrence in the mandible. There is no racial or sexual predilection and it is rarely diagnosed in individuals younger than 6 years of age. Clinically, the involved tooth is vital and asymptomatic. However, it is notable that there often is a history of trauma to the tooth. Hypercementosis is frequently associated with systemic disorders such as giantism, acromegaly or Paget's disease. A synonym is *cementum hyperplasia*.

Taurodont tooth (Fig. W15)

Taurodont tooth describes any tooth that congenitally develops a large body and pulp chamber, with very little root formation and an overall tooth size that is normal. Children under 6 years of age are rarely affected. The pulp chamber of a taurodont tooth is gradually obliterated as the patient's age increases. A synonym includes *bull-like tooth*.

Turner's tooth (Fig. W16)

A *Turner's tooth* refers to an enamel hypoplasia of a permanent tooth that is believed to originate from a precursory, periapically involved, deciduous tooth. This typically occurs in the anterior regions of the maxilla and the mandible. Clinically, Turner's tooth manifests in varying degrees of severity. The tooth may vary from simply being stained to, in severe cases, only a shell of a tooth being present. There is no racial or sexual predilection. The appearance of the affected tooth varies according to the severity of the lesion. Typically, the crown of a Turner's tooth has irregular contours, and its root occasionally has an irregular outline. Its size is also quite variable, depending upon the severity of the lesion. A synonym is *localized hypoplasia*.

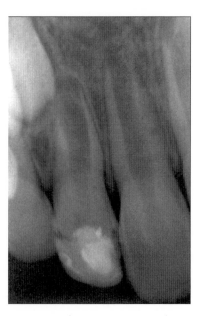

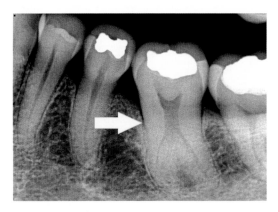

Fig. W15 Taurodontism.

Fig. W16 Turner's tooth. (Source: Courtesy of P. R. Ritwick.)

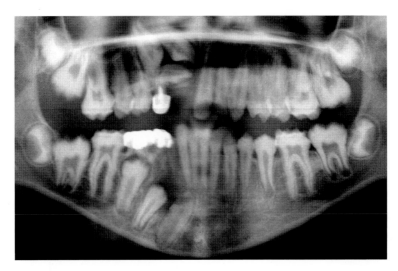

Fig. W17 Amelogenesis imperfecta (e.g. enamel hypoplasia).

Developmental factors

Amelogenesis imperfecta (Fig. W17)

Amelogenesis imperfecta represents a developmental anomaly of enamel. Two basic types of amelogenesis imperfecta exist: *enamel hypoplasia* and *enamel hypocalcification*. Neither type shows any racial or sexual predilection. It may be present in either the deciduous or the permanent dentitions. In the hypoplastic type, there is a reduction in the thickness of enamel. The crowns of teeth often appear square because they are devoid of normal mesial and distal contours. However, the radiologic density of a hypoplastic tooth appears normal. In the hypocalcified type, the enamel is of proper thickness but it is not properly calcified. The resultant appearance is a tooth with proper contours and an enamel layer that is more radiolucent than normal. This is made apparent by the lack of image contrast between the enamel and dentin. Clinically, both types often show a discoloration of the crowns, ranging from yellow to brown, and there frequently is marked attrition of the involved teeth. Synonyms include *hereditary enamel dysplasia, hereditary brown enamel, hereditary brown opalescent teeth, hereditary enamel hypoplasia, hereditary enamel hypocalcification* and *enamel dysplasia*.

Dentinal dysplasia (Fig. W18)

Dentinal dysplasia is a disturbance in dentin formation of one or more teeth, characterized by little or no pulp chambers and very little root formation. Both the deciduous and permanent dentitions may be affected. Clinically, the teeth appear normal in morphology and color, but they often become loose and are exfoliated prematurely. There is no age, sex or racial predilection. A synonym is *rootless teeth*.

Dentinogenesis imperfecta (Fig. W19)

Dentinogenesis imperfecta refers to a developmental anomaly of dentin formation found in both the deciduous and permanent dentitions. There is no sexual or racial predilection and it may be diagnosed in any age group. The teeth are frequently described as "tulip teeth," because they often have thin, short roots and constricted

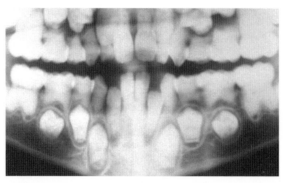

A

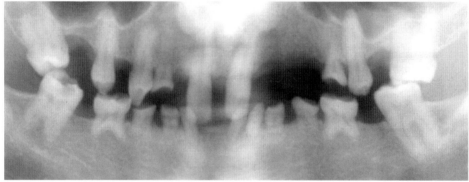

B

Fig. W18 Dentinal dysplasia.

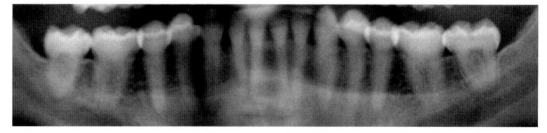

Fig. W19 Dentinogenesis imperfecta. (Source: Courtesy of Dr. J. Townsend.)

necks, which gives the crowns a bulbous shape. Initially, the pulp chambers are wide, but gradually there is a partial or total precocious obliteration of the pulp chambers as a result of continued dentin formation. Clinically, the teeth often have a translucent or opalescent hue and marked attrition. Synonyms include *hereditary opalescent dentin* and *opalescent dentin*.

Hypoplasia, enamel

Enamel hypoplasia is the incomplete or defective formation of the enamel matrix of teeth. Its etiology may be either hereditary or environmental and one or more deciduous or permanent teeth may be affected. The patient's dental and medical histories may indicate possible etiologic factors such as a nutritional deficiency, metabolic disorders, childhood diseases or excessive fluoride intake. There is no sexual or racial predilection and it may be diagnosed in any age group. The clinical appearance of hypoplasia may vary from a slight discoloration to severe pitting and irregularity in the shape of a crown. The tooth appears normal except for a reduced thickness and, possibly, an irregular outline of its crown. (see Amelogenesis imperfecta). Synonyms include *mottled tooth, enamel dysplasia, hereditary enamel hypoplasia* and *brown teeth*.

Odontoma, complex (Fig. W20)

A *complex odontoma* is an odontogenic tumor composed of an irregular conglomerate mass of dental tissues which bears no resemblance to a tooth. Typically it is a slow-growing lesion, varying in size from a few millimeters to several centimeters in diameter. Any tooth-bearing areas of the maxilla or mandible may be affected. However, it is most often located in the mandibular molar regions. Controversy, similar to that surrounding the compound odontoma, still exists regarding the etiology of this lesion. The average patient is between 5 and 30 years of age, but it may be evident in any age group. Also, there is no racial or sexual predilection. The complex odontoma appears typically as a unilocular radiolucency with smooth contours, within which are numerous patternless radiopacities. This often gives it the appearance of being surrounded by a radiolucent capsule. In addition, the borders of the lesion are usually scalloped and radiopaque. The patient often presents with a painless swelling. A synonym is *complex composite odontome*.

Odontoma, compound (Fig. W21)

A *compound odontoma* is an odontogenic tumor composed of one or more supernumerary denticles of different sizes and shapes.

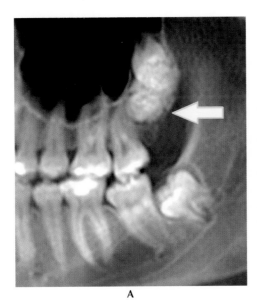
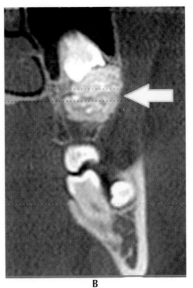

A   B

Fig. W20 Complex odontoma. A. Sagittal view. B. Coronal cross-sectional view of the same tooth as A.

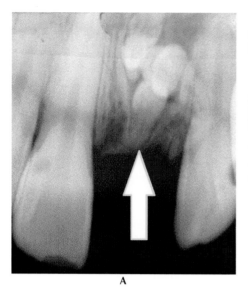

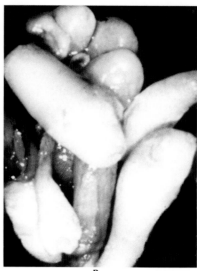

A   B

Fig. W21 Compound odontoma.

Typically, it is a single, slow-growing lesion, varying in size from a few millimeters to several centimeters in diameter. Any tooth-bearing areas of the maxilla or mandible may be affected. However, it is most often located in the maxillary central incisor region, followed by the mandibular molar region. Interestingly, these are areas that show a predisposition for supernumerary teeth. However, controversy still exists concerning the etiology of the lesion, with suggestions that local trauma, infection or excessive budding of the dental lamina may lead to development of the odontoma. The average patient is between 5 and 30 years of age, but it may be diagnosed in all age groups. Also, there is no racial or sexual predilection. The compound odontoma typically appears as a unilocular radiolucency, within which are well-defined tooth-like radiopacities. This gives the lesion the impression of being surrounded by a radiolucent capsule. In addition, the borders of the lesion are often scalloped and radiopaque. Clinically, the patient often presents with a painless swelling. Synonyms include *compound composite odontome* and *cystic compound composite odontome*.

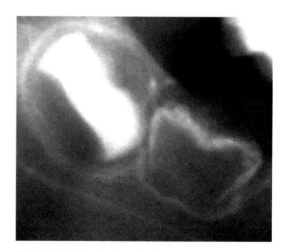

Fig. W22 Regional odontodysplasia.

Odontodysplasia, regional (Fig. W22)

Regional odontodysplasia is a developmental anomaly in which one or more teeth in a localized area of the maxilla and/or the mandible have exceedingly large pulp chambers and very thin layers of enamel and dentin. Both the enamel and dentin show a marked reduction in density. As well, the trabeculae in the affected region appear very fine. It is notable that the size of the affected teeth is either normal or slightly smaller than average. The maxillary teeth are more commonly involved than those in the mandible and the most frequently affected teeth are those in the anterior region. There is no racial or sexual predilection and it may be diagnosed in all age categories. Clinically, the patient may present with delayed or unerupted teeth. Synonyms include *odontogenesis imperfecta, odontodysplasia, odontogenic dysplasia* and *ghost teeth.*

Osteogenesis imperfecta

Osteogenesis imperfecta is a disease of bone characterized by extreme fragility and porosity of the bones, blue sclera, deafness and an unusual shape of the skull. It usually is present at birth or manifests itself shortly afterwards. There is no racial or sexual predilection. The oral manifestations are identical to dentinogenesis imperfecta, although there are cases in which the teeth appear normal. It is notable that osteogenesis imperfecta is usually diagnosed by a medical doctor, prior to the patient's first dental appointment. Synonyms include *brittle bones, fragilitas ossium, osteopsathyrosis* and *Lobstein's disease.*

Pulpal obliteration (Fig. W23)

Pulpal obliteration refers to the partial or total constriction of the pulp chamber and/or root canal of a tooth. Any number of permanent or deciduous teeth may be affected and there is no age, sex or racial predilection. It appears as a generalized pacification of the pulp. Clinically, the patient is often asymptomatic, but pulpal obliteration is often associated with trauma or developmental disorders such as dentinogenesis imperfecta.

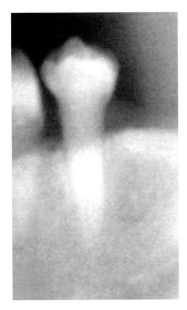

Fig. W23 Pulpal obliteration.

Environmental factors

Abrasion (Fig. W24)

Abrasion is the pathologic wearing down of a tooth structure by mechanical means. The amount of wear is variable, ranging from under a millimeter to total destruction of the crown of a tooth. The area of abrasion appears more radiolucent than the remainder of the crown and it often has irregular borders. Abrasion may be associated with any deciduous or permanent teeth, and there is no age, sex or racial predilection. Various etiologic factors include improper toothbrushing technique, abrasive dentifrice, ill-fitting partial dentures, personal habits or occupational hazards. The patient is often asymptomatic.

Ankylosis (Fig. W25)

Ankylosis of a tooth is the proliferation of bone between the alveolar bone and the cementum or dentin of a tooth, with the elimination of any

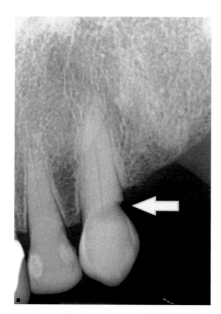

Fig. W24 Tooth abrasion: caused by a partial denture clasp.

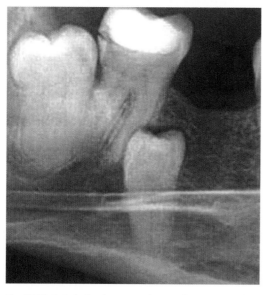

Fig. W25 Ankylosis of unerupted premolar.

intervening soft tissue. Its etiology is uncertain, but there often is a history of trauma to or infection in the tooth. There is no racial or sexual predilection and it may be diagnosed in all age groups. Although the deciduous molars are primarily

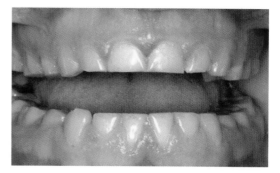

Fig. W26 Attrition. (Source: Courtesy of R. Saeves.)

affected, it may involve any deciduous or permanent teeth. The normal radiolucent periodontal ligament space is transformed into a radiopaque region confluent with the surrounding bone. Occasionally, the root may have an irregular outline and a *moth-eaten appearance* ☢. As a result, there may also be a reduction in the overall size of the tooth. Clinically, the affected tooth is generally asymptomatic.

Attrition (Fig. W26)

Attrition is the physiologic or pathologic wearing down of a tooth structure as a result of tooth to tooth contact. The amount of tooth reduction is variable, ranging from under a millimeter to total destruction of the crown of the tooth. Typically, the pattern of wear is irregular. In addition to the reduction in the size of the tooth, pulpal obliteration may also be apparent. Attrition may be associated with any deciduous or permanent teeth and there is no age, sex or racial predilection. Etiologic factors associated with pathologic attrition include occupations where a patient is exposed to abrasive airborne materials, malpositioned teeth or a coarse diet. The patient is often asymptomatic.

Calculus (Fig. W27)

Calculus is a hard mineralized deposit found only above the bone level around one or more

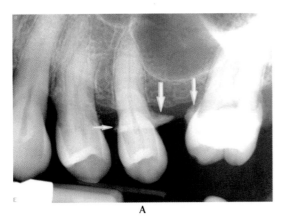

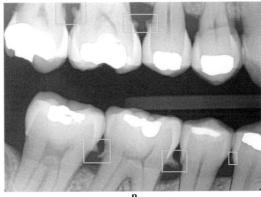

A   B

Fig. W27 Calculus.

deciduous or permanent teeth. There is no sexual or racial predilection and it is found in all age groups. Calculus usually appears as a spur-like projection near the cervical aspect of a tooth or as a linear radiopaque line running from the mesial to distal aspects of a tooth. However, in the case of a heavy build-up of calculus, it may appear as a wide continuous radiopaque band adjoining several teeth. Clinically, calculus varies in color from yellow to dark brown or black, depending upon the amount of stain present. The patient may complain of bad breath, loose teeth and bleeding gums. As well, the patient often claims that his or her teeth are chipping or breaking. Synonyms include *tartar* and *calcareous deposit*.

Caries, dental

See Section V.

Erosion (Fig. W28)

Erosion is the pathologic wearing down of a tooth structure by chemical means. The amount of wear is variable, ranging from under a millimeter to total destruction of the crown. The area of erosion appears more radiolucent than

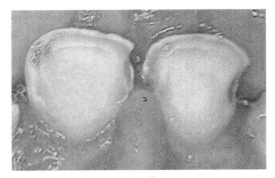

Fig. W28 Erosion.

the remainder of the crown and it often has well-defined borders. Erosion may affect any deciduous or permanent teeth and there is no age, sex or racial predilection. It is notable that the mesial and distal surfaces of teeth are rarely affected. Clinically, the affected area often appears as either a smoothly polished, disc-shaped cavity or as a pitted tooth surface. Various etiologic factors include occupational hazards, diet, medications or a low salivary pH value.

Foreign body (Fig. W29)

A *foreign body* is any object or particle of material that is not indigenous to the area in which it is located. Foreign bodies may be any shape and size, but they must be radiopaque. They may occur anywhere within an x-ray image and there is no age, sex or racial predilection. Clinically, the patient may present with pain and swelling in the affected area and its etiology

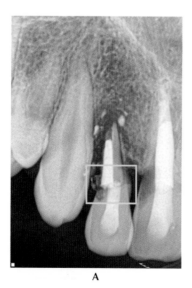

Fig. W29 Bullet fragments.

may be ascertained from a history of previous trauma or dental treatment.

Fracture (Fig. W30)

Fracture of a crown or root of a tooth is a common injury, often a result of a sudden severe trauma. Other etiologic factors include large dental restorations, internal resorption and endodontic treatment. One or more deciduous and/or permanent teeth in either the maxilla or mandible may be fractured. There is no racial predilection, but fractures occur more frequently in the anterior teeth of children because of the greater incidence of trauma in such individuals. A fracture is evident when there is a discontinuity in the outline of a tooth, but there may or may not be displacement of any part of the fractured tooth. A root fracture often appears as a regular or irregular radiolucent line. However, depending on the angle of a fracture, it may or may not be visible on every x-ray image. A crown fracture also may not be visible on an x-ray image. The border outline

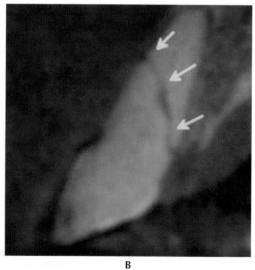

A   B

Fig. W30 Root fractures. (B. Source: Courtesy of Drs M. Beilman, M. Burns and G. Klasser.)

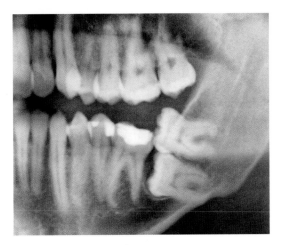

Fig. W31 Impaction: molars.

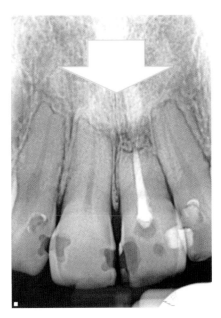

Fig. W32 External resorption.

may be regular or irregular. Clinically, the tooth may be sensitive to temperature changes, painful to percussion or loose. A CBCT may reveal a fracture line.

Impaction (Fig. W31)

An *impacted tooth* is any partially or totally unerupted tooth that is prevented from normal eruption by an obstruction. Clinically, there is no age, sex or racial predilection. However, the patient may experience *pericoronitis* ☢.

Resorption, external (Fig. W32)

External resorption is the destruction of a crown and/or root of a deciduous or permanent tooth originating at the outer surface and continuing pulpally. This results in either a smooth or an irregular periphery. There is a reduction in its size that can vary from a millimeter to total destruction of the tooth. Its etiology may reflect normal physiologic resorption, previous orthodontic treatment, trauma, an apicoectomy, an artifact or a congenital defect. There is no sexual or racial predilection and it may be diagnosed in any age group.

Resorption, internal (Fig. W33)

Internal resorption is the destruction of dentin commencing from the pulp chamber and continuing outwards. Although it may affect either the deciduous or permanent dentition, it primarily is found within permanent teeth. Internal resorption generally results in a well-defined round or oval radiolucent area in the central portion of a tooth, associated with the pulp chamber and occasionally extending to the external surface of the root. However, the resorbed area may assume any shape and its size may range from a millimeter to total destruction of the tooth. There is no racial or sexual predilection and it may be diagnosed in any age group. It is noteworthy that there often is a history of a pulpotomy or other trauma to

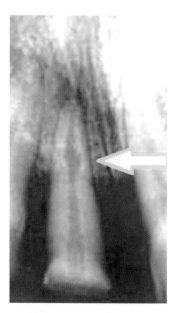

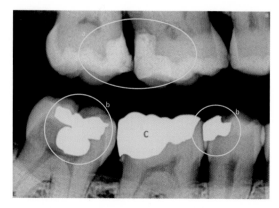

Fig. W34 Restorations: a, composite restorations; b, amalgam restorations; c, *onlay restoration* ☢.

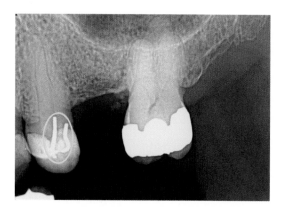

Fig. W35 Pin associated with restoration.

Fig. W33 Internal resorption. (Source: Courtesy of M. Fernandes.)

the affected tooth. Clinically, the tooth characteristically has a pink color. Synonyms include *pink spot*, *internal granuloma*, *chronic perforation* and *hyperplasia of pulp*.

Restorations, dental

Dental restorations encompass a diverse range of clinical and radiological appearances. There is no characteristic location, number or shape, and there is no age, sex or racial predilection. As well, the size of a restoration is quite variable, ranging from a couple of millimeters in diameter to total involvement of a crown. Composite restorations often match the natural shade of tooth structure and may be overlooked in a clinical examination. A composite restoration appears as either a well-defined radiopaque or radiolucent area within the coronal portion of a tooth (Figs W34, W35, W36 and W37). Porcelain restorations are similar to composites (Fig. W38). Metallic restorations, such as amalgam and gold appear as well-defined radiopaque areas and they are primarily located within posterior teeth (Figs W39 and W40). Gutta percha (Fig. W38) is a radiopaque filling material found within a root canal. Typically, it will appear as a conical shape in the pulpal portion of a tooth, extending from the coronal portion of a tooth to its apex. Figures W41, W42, W43 and W44 illustrate other restoration features.

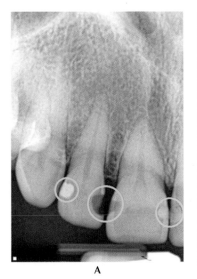
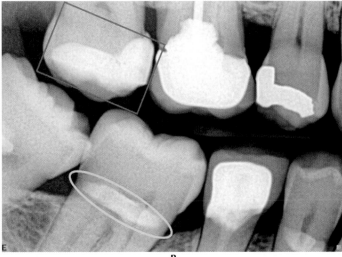

A B

Fig. W36 Class III composite restorations. A. Composite material with radiopaque filler and those without radiopaque filler that appear radiolucent. B. Highlighted cervical composite on the mandibular first molar and mesio-occlusal composite on the maxillary second molar.

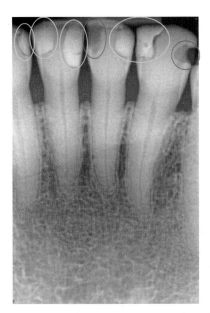

Fig. W37 Composite restorations: red circles, composite material without radiopaque filler; yellow circles, composite with radiopaque filler.

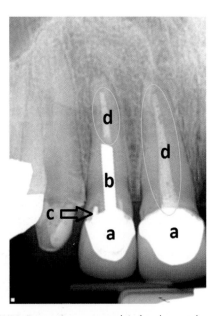

Fig. W38 Restorations: a, porcelain fused to metal crowns; b, prefabricated post; c, pin; d. gutta percha.

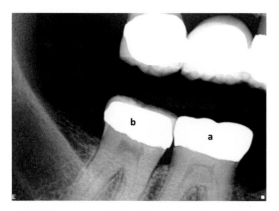

Fig. W39 Crowns: a, full gold crown on the mandibular first molar; b, porcelain bonded to metal crown on the mandibular second molar.

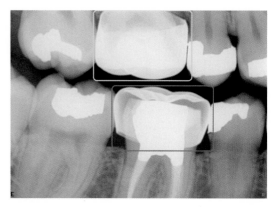

Fig. W40 Stainless steel crowns on the maxillary and mandibular first molars.

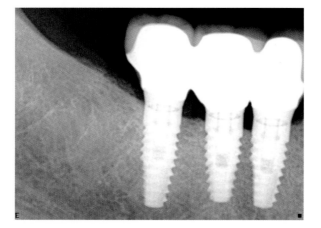

Fig. W41 Implants.

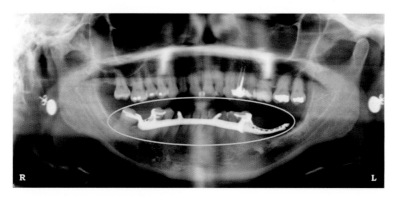

Fig. W42 Cast of a removable partial denture (circled).

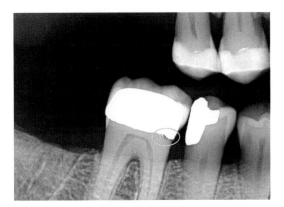

Fig. W43 Open margin with the crown, recurrent decay or radiolucent cement? A clinical assessment would be necessary to determine.

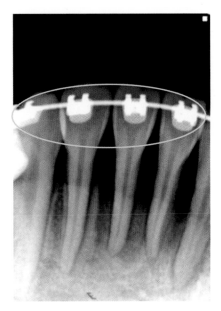

Fig. W44 Orthodontic hardware.

X

Osseous Pathology (Alphabetic)

Explanatory note: First of all, this book is not intended to be a comprehensive atlas of oral pathology. As mentioned earlier, most dental textbooks only show dental images of osseous pathology during a classic late stage of development which often stereotypes their appearances. The problem is that an osseous lesion will often appear dramatically different in earlier stages of development when most patients may be unaware of any problem and something is incidentally observed on a dental x-ray image. Unlike most dental anomalies, the size, shape, borders, loculations and even density of an osseous lesion may be dramatically different dependent upon the time of discovery. A large soap bubble radiolucency initially began as a pinpoint, unilocular radiolucency. A radiopaque lesion may have transitioned from a radiolucency through a mixed phase until it progressed into a radiopacity. This is analogous to comparing photographs of an adult person and assuming that the individual appeared physically similar as a newborn and throughout childhood. Consequently, only written descriptions of the osseous entities will be found here. A review of the terminology used to describe osseous pathology will be found in Appendix 4.

Abscess, periapical

A *periapical abscess* is an acute or chronic suppurative lesion affecting either the deciduous or permanent dentition. It may be single or multiple in number and the size of the lesion varies from a few millimeters to a couple of centimeters in diameter. The periapical abscess occurs in all age groups and there is no racial or sexual predilection. Typically, there is a history of caries or trauma to the affected tooth and the duration may be years before the abscess is diagnosed. It appears as a unilocular, diffuse or well-circumscribed radiolucent area at the apex of a tooth. It is notable, however, that there is no radiopaque border around the lesion. During the acute stage, the patient often complains of pain, swelling, tenderness to percussion, a slight extrusion of the affected tooth from the tooth socket and, occasionally, a fever. During the chronic stage, the affected tooth is often asymptomatic, but there usually is suppuration from an opening of a fistulous tract to the oral cavity. In both stages, the affected tooth is nonvital. Synonyms include *acute alveolar abscess*, *dento-alveolar abscess*, *alveolar abscess* and *acute rarefying osteitis*.

Fundamentals of Oral and Maxillofacial Radiology, First Edition. J. Sean Hubar.
© 2017 John Wiley & Sons, Inc. Published 2017 by John Wiley & Sons, Inc.
Companion website: www.wiley.com/go/hubar/radiology

Ameloblastoma

An *ameloblastoma* is a benign odontogenic neoplasm of epithelial origin. The average patient is between 30 and 50 years of age when the tumor is diagnosed, but it may occur in patients of all ages. It has been generally accepted that there is no racial or sexual predilection. Trauma, infection or previous dental extractions have been cited in numerous cases. On average, the duration of time between the patient's first awareness of the lesion and the diagnosis of the ameloblastoma is over 2 years. Ameloblastomas typically are single in number and found in the posterior (i.e. molar–ramus) regions of the mandible. The size of the lesion is quite variable, ranging from a 0.5 cm to over 18 cm in diameter. However, the average size is from 3 to 5 cm in diameter. A larger ameloblastoma often will appear as a multilocular radiolucent lesion with a *soap bubble appearance* ☢ (Fig. X1). Regardless of size, it still may be a unilocular radiolucency. The border is also quite variable depending upon the stage of development at the time of the diagnosis. Early in its development, the ameloblastoma displays well-defined borders without any expansion of the cortical plate. Later stages reveal a lesion with a notching and/or undulating expansion of the cortical plate and ill-defined borders. Careful histologic examination is required as an ameloblastoma frequently may arise in the wall of a dentigerous cyst. The ameloblastoma has also been found to develop in association with a fibroma and/or an odontoma. Clinically, the ameloblastoma is often observed as a painless swelling of the mandible. Synonyms include *adamantinoma* and *central epithelioma*.

Antrolith

An *antrolith* is a mass that arises from the deposition of calcific salts around the nuclei of blood, mucous or foreign bodies. The antrolith is a generalized term simply used to indicate that

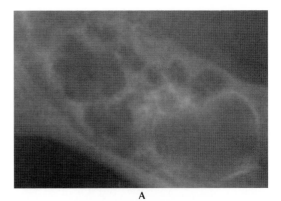

A

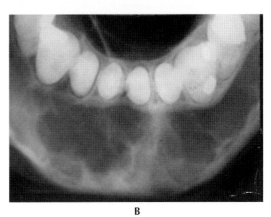

B

Fig. X1 A. Multilocular. B. Soap bubble appearance.

the mass is found within an antrum. It may be single or multiple in number and they may vary from a few millimeters to a few centimeters in size. They are most commonly found in individuals younger than 40 years of age, but they may occur in any age group. Also, there is no sexual or racial predilection. Antroliths appear as regular or irregular radiopacities with well-defined margins. The patient's past medical and dental histories often reveal an incident of an earlier traumatic extraction or an instance during childhood when a small object (e.g. cherry pit) was inserted into the patient's nose. Antroliths are slow-growing lesions and the individual may not be cognizant of any unusual symptoms for years. Some patients may complain of headaches, nasal obstruction and/or discharge, laryngitis or epistaxis, while other individuals may be totally asymptomatic. Of note, similar calcifications located within the nose are called *rhinoliths* or *nasal calculi*.

Bone marrow defect

A *bone marrow defect* develops when foci of hematopoietic or fibro-fatty marrow form a localized collection of large marrow spaces. The etiology remains unknown, but it is often associated with chronic anemia. The condyle, the angle of the mandible and the maxillary tuberosity are the most frequently affected sites. The typical patient is white, female and 30–50 years of age at the time of diagnosis. However, it may be found in either sex and in any race. The bone marrow defect may be single or multiple in number and it ranges from a few millimeters to several centimeters in diameter. It is quite variable in appearance, often appearing as a poorly defined radiolucency with irregular borders. Occasionally, it may appear as a sharply defined radiolucency. The bone marrow defect is usually asymptomatic and it is often discovered inadvertently during routine radiologic examination.

Calcifying epithelial odontogenic tumor

A *calcifying epithelial odontogenic tumor (CEOT)* is a slow-growing benign neoplasm found only within the maxilla and mandible. The tumor is predominantly located within the premolar–molar regions, with the mandible being more frequently affected than the maxilla. Typically it is a single lesion, varying from 2 to 5 cm in size. There is no racial or sexual predilection and while the average patient is 30–60 years of age at the time of diagnosis, it may be found in all age groups. The calcifying epithelial odontogenic tumor is quite variable. Initially, it may appear as a well-defined or diffuse unilocular or multilocular radiolucency often around the coronal aspect of a fully embedded tooth. The late stage of a CEOT is characterized by the formation of multiple, small, radiopaque foci within the radiolucency. Clinically it presents as a painless swelling of long duration, varying from weeks to several years prior to the patient seeking dental care. A synonym is *Pindborg tumor*.

Cementoblastoma

A *cementoblastoma* is a benign neoplasm consisting of sheets of cementum-like tissue, which may not be mineralized at the periphery of the mass or in the more active growth areas. However, there is a paucity of precise information available to distinguish this lesion clearly from periapical osseous dysplasia. Typically, the cementoblastoma is a single, slow-growing lesion found only in the tooth-bearing areas of the maxilla and mandible. Classically, it is attached to the root of the mandibular first molar and the average size of the lesion is 1 cm in diameter. There is a predilection for males, whose average age is 25 years, but it may be found in any age group and there is no racial predilection. The cementoblastoma appears as a mottled, dense radiopaque mass bordered by a well-demarcated peripheral radiolucent zone, confluent with one or more roots that may show evidence of root resorption. Clinically, the cementoblastoma often presents as an expansion of the bone and there may or may not be pain associated with it. Synonyms include *true cementoblastoma* and *benign cementoblastoma*.

Cherubism

Cherubism is a rare fibrous proliferating disease found only within the maxilla and/or the mandible. There is no racial predilection, but males are more frequently affected. It is notable that the majority of cases occur in childhood, with the average patient being between 2 and 5 years of age. Also, a natural regression of the lesion occurs as the patient approaches puberty, often leading to a near normal appearance by the time the patient is 20 years of age. Cherubism is generally accepted to be a hereditary disorder and examination of the parents' past medical histories will often confirm a familial history of the disease. Cherubism usually appears as a well-defined, multiloculated radiolucency having a *soap bubble* appearance. Occasionally, it appears as a unilocular radiolucency. In addition, it typically occurs bilaterally in the posterior regions of the mandible and results in osseous expansion and thinning of the cortical plate. While in the maxilla, the lesions may be found predominantly in the tuberosity areas. The healed bone generally appears to be abnormally calcified or sclerotic. Clinically, the patient presents with a painless, symmetric, bony hard enlargement of the mandible and/or the maxilla, giving rise to the chubby face suggestive of a cherub. Synonyms include *familial fibrous dysplasia of the jaws, disseminated juvenile fibrous dysplasia, familial multilocular cystic disease of the jaws* and *familial fibrous swelling of the jaws*.

Condensing osteitis

Condensing osteitis is a chronic inflammatory process within the tooth-bearing areas of the maxilla and mandible that results in a localized area of bone formation. Typically, it is a single lesion occurring in the premolar–molar regions of the mandible. The associated tooth is carious or has a large restoration. It is most frequently found in young adults, but it can also be diagnosed in older individuals. The average size of the lesion is from 0.5 to 1.5 cm in diameter. Because the lesion is slow growing and usually asymptomatic, the patient may not be cognizant of the condition. The lesion can be classified into early and late stages. The early stage is characterized by a region of dense osteosclerosis having rounded and lobulated margins with either well-defined or diffuse borders. The late

stage shows the same lesion with a radiolucent rim and often there is expansion of the alveolar bone. It is notable that the lesion appears outside of the lamina dura. Synonyms include *focal sclerosing osteomyelitis, enostosis, sclerosing osteitis, bone whorl* and *osseous dysplasia*.

Cysts

Aneurysmal bone cyst

An *aneurysmal bone cyst* is a controversial lesion of bone, which has been considered to be a variant of the giant cell tumor. Essentially, the aneurysmal bone cyst is a solitary, localized and expanded fibrous lesion honeycombed by an enormously plexiform vascular bed. The typical patient is under 20 years of age at the time of diagnosis, yet it may be present in any age group. Males are more frequently affected, but there is no apparent racial predilection. Characteristically, it is a rapidly growing lesion located within the long bones and vertebrae with rare cases found in the posterior regions of the mandible and maxilla. While the etiology is uncertain, there often is a history of trauma to the area. It typically appears as a unilocular radiolucency (Fig. X2). However, it may be a multiloculated radiolucency with a *soap bubble* appearance (Fig. X1). In either situation, the margins may or may not be well-defined and the cortical plate often is expanded and perforated. Clinically, the aneurysmal bone cyst presents as a swelling with or without pain, *paresthesia* ♣♠ and tooth displacement. Synonyms include *ossifying hematoma, aneurysmal giant cell tumor, subperiosteal giant cell tumor* and *periosteal benign giant cell tumor*.

Botryoid odontogenic cyst

The *botryoid* ♣♠ *odontogenic cyst (BOC)* is a polycystic variant of the lateral periodontal cyst. The age group ranges from 23 to 85 years. A BOC is typically multilocular (Fig. X1) and is larger than a lateral periodontal cyst, ranging

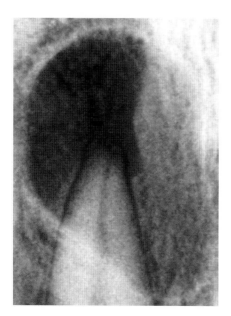

Fig. X2 Unilocular appearance.

between 0.5 and 4.5 cm in diameter. The BOC often extends into the periapical region of involved teeth. It can be asymptomatic or very painful. Paresthesia and *tumefaction* ☢ have also been reported. Although the histopathologic features of BOCs are similar to lateral periodontal cysts, the BOC recurrence rate is higher.

Calcifying odontogenic cyst

A *calcifying odontogenic cyst (COC)* is an unusual lesion, manifesting some features of both cysts and solid neoplasms. It presents as a slow-growing, single lesion that ranges from 1 to 10 cm in diameter. Predominantly, it is located within the posterior regions of the mandible and, less frequently, it is found within the maxilla. There is no racial or sexual predilection, although the majority of cases occur in adulthood. The COC is quite variable. It may be a well-defined or ill-defined, unilocular or multilocular radiolucency (Figs X1 and X2) There will be varying numbers of small radiopaque masses within the radiolucency. As well, it is often associated with an unerupted tooth.

Clinically, the patient often presents with a painless swelling. Synonyms include *calcifying cystic odontogenic tumor* and *Gorlin cyst*.

Dentigerous cyst

A *dentigerous cyst* is odontogenic in origin, arising from the enamel organ after partial completion of the crown of the tooth. The incidence is primarily in the posterior region of the mandible around the third molar. Occasionally they have been diagnosed in the maxilla, around which the cuspid and bicuspids are most frequently involved. A dentigerous cyst may be located either on the coronal or lateral aspect of an unerupted tooth. Typically, it is slow-growing lesion ranging from a couple of millimeters to several centimeters in diameter. There does not appear to be any racial or sexual predilection. The average patient is between 10 and 20 years of age at the time of diagnosis, but it may found in any age group. A dentigerous cyst predominantly appears as a single, oval or round, unilocular radiolucency with well-defined margins (Fig. X2). It may or may not have a radiopaque rim. The radiolucency is devoid of any internal trabeculation or calcifications. Occasionally, it may appear as a multiloculated radiolucency (Fig. X1) and display an aggressive behavior leading to bony expansion, root resorption and displacement of teeth. Clinically, the patient is often asymptomatic, but may be cognizant of a missing tooth or delayed tooth eruption. A synonym is the *follicular cyst*.

Incisive canal cyst

An *incisive canal cyst* is a non-odontogenic cyst that originates from the proliferation of the epithelial remnants of the nasopalatine duct. Its etiology is unknown, but various factors, such as trauma and bacterial infection, have been proposed to explain its development. It is a single entity found only in the area of the incisive canal or the anterior palatine papilla. Although it may be found in all age categories, there is prevalence for individuals between 30 and 50 years of age. There is no racial predilection, but males are primarily affected. The incisive canal cyst appears as a well-defined, round, ovoid or heart-shaped radiolucency (Fig. X2). The average size of the lesion ranges from under 0.5 to 1 cm in diameter. The incisive canal cyst is usually asymptomatic, but it occasionally presents as a painful fluctuant swelling. Synonyms include *median anterior maxillary cyst*, *anterior palatine foramen cyst* and *nasopalatine duct cyst*.

Keratocystic odontogenic tumor

Keratocystic odontogenic tumor is an all-encompassing term used to describe any cyst that is derived from epithelium associated with the development of the dental structures. Typically, an odontogenic cyst is a single lesion, with less than 10% of the patients presenting with multiple cysts. A preponderance of the cases involves the posterior regions of the mandible, but it may be located anywhere within either the maxilla or the mandible. The size of the cyst is quite variable, ranging from 1 cm to over 7 cm in diameter. While there is a predilection for males, particularly in those under 30 years of age, it may occur in all age groups of either sex. The patient's dental records often reveal the etiology of the cyst, as it is usually associated with a history of tooth extraction, an inadequately treated cyst or missing and unerupted teeth. Characteristically, the appearance of an odontogenic cyst is a well-defined round or oval unilocular radiolucency with smooth borders (Fig. X2). Other features may include a multiloculated appearance (Fig. X1), scalloped borders, thinning and expansion of the cortical plate and root displacement with or without root resorption. It may or may not have a corticated (i.e. radiopaque) border. Clinically, the odontogenic cyst is usually asymptomatic. However, a cyst of long duration may cause pain and swelling of the jaw. A synonym is an *odontogenic keratocyst*.

Lateral periodontal cyst

A *lateral periodontal cyst (LPC)* is a non-inflammatory and non-keratinized developmental cyst located lateral to the root of a vital tooth. They arise either between the roots or along the lateral periodontium of vital erupted teeth. A LPC typically appears as a well-defined round or ovoid unilocular radiolucency located along the root between the alveolar crest and apex of the tooth. The average size is less than 1 cm in diameter. Occasionally, there may be a divergence of adjacent roots and loss of the lamina dura. Histopathologic examination is necessary to differentiate a LPC from other odontogenic cysts (see Botryoid odontogenic cyst).

Median palatine cyst

A *median palatine cyst* is a fissural cyst that arises from epithelium trapped along the line of fusion of the palatal processes. The cyst is a single lesion found posterior to the anterior palatine papilla, in the midline of the hard palate. There is no racial or sexual predilection and it may be found in all age categories. However, there is prevalence for persons aged 30–50 years. It appears as a well-defined unilocular, round or oval radiolucency with or without a radiopaque periphery (Fig. X2). The average size of the lesion is 2 cm in diameter. Clinically, the median palatine cyst usually presents as a painless swelling, but it occasionally causes discomfort.

Periapical cyst

A *periapical cyst* arises from a non-vital tooth. It is the most common variety of cyst found in the mandible and maxilla. Similar to the periapical abscess, it may be single or multiple in number. The size of the cyst varies from a centimeter to multiple centimeters in diameter. The periapical cyst occurs in all age groups but is more commonly found in the third to sixth decades of life. It can be found in both sexes, but is slightly more common in males. Typically, there is a history of deep caries or trauma to the affected tooth that results in necrosis of the pulp. It often is non-symptomatic and found incidentally on x-ray images. A periapical cyst typically appears as a single, uniform, well-defined radiolucency with or without a cortical border (Fig. X2). Unless it is affected by surrounding structures, it typically appears round. Large cysts may cause expansion of the surrounding cortical plates, displace adjacent teeth and cause root resorption. Treatment often entails endodontic therapy, apical surgery or extraction of the offending tooth with enucleation of the cyst. If there was incomplete removal of the cyst when the tooth was extracted, the resultant lesion is now referred to as a *residual cyst* ☢. Synonyms include *radicular cyst*, *dental cyst* and *periapical periodontal cyst*.

Stafne bone cyst

A *Stafne bone cyst* is generally accepted to be a salivary gland tissue inclusion defect that occurs during the development and growth of the mandible. It often is an incidental finding on panoramic images. The lesion is always situated between the mandibular canal and the cortical plate and, typically, in the region of the first molar and angle of the mandible. Occasionally, it may be located in the central incisor and bicuspid region. As well, there is a growing consensus of opinion that the lesion connects to the surrounding soft tissues. Males are primarily affected, but there is no racial predilection. It often appears as a single, round or oval unilocular radiolucency with either well-defined or ill-defined borders (see Fig. Y16). The size of the lesion averages from 1 to 3 cm in diameter. On occasion, it has been reported to occur bilaterally. Clinically, the lesion is usually asymptomatic and, therefore, tends to be discovered inadvertently during routine radiologic examination. To rule out any pathology, a CBCT scan is best for diagnosing this defect. Synonyms include *Stafne bone cavity*, *developmental lingual mandibular salivary gland depression*, *static bone cavity, static bone cyst, idiopathic bone cavity, lingual mandibular bone cavity* and *latent bone cyst*.

Traumatic bone cyst

A *traumatic bone cyst* is a controversial lesion. The general consensus is that this lesion lacks an epithelial lining and therefore the term "cyst" is a misnomer. It is most frequently located in the long bones and in the posterior regions of the mandible, lying above the mandibular canal. Although it can occur in any bone, it rarely is found in the maxilla. The typical patient is male and between 10 and 20 years of age at the time of diagnosis. However, it can be found in any age group of either sex and there is no racial predilection. While the etiology of this lesion remains unknown, there is often a history of trauma to the involved area. The traumatic bone cyst is a slow-growing lesion. Consequently, the patient may not be cognizant of the lesion existing, sometimes for several years. A traumatic bone cyst frequently appears as a lobulated, fairly well-demarcated unilocular radiolucency (Fig. X2) extending high up between the roots of teeth. Typically, there will be trabeculae found within the radiolucency and the teeth in the area will be vital. Clinically, the traumatic bone cyst often presents as a painful swelling, but occasionally it may be totally asymptomatic. Synonyms include *intraosseous hematoma, blood cyst, hemorrhagic cyst, solitary bone cyst, simple bone cyst, progressive bone cavity, extravasation cyst* and *unicameral cyst*.

Exostosis

An *exostosis* is a benign osseous growth characterized as a bony excrescence on the outer surface of a bone. Intraorally, the exostosis predominantly occurs in the posterior regions of either the maxilla or the mandible. Typically, it averages from 1 to 2 cm in size and it may be either single or multiple in number. Although the exostosis may arise at any age, it seems to be somewhat more common in young adults. There is no sexual predilection. The exostosis generally appears as a rounded radiopaque mass with a well-circumscribed lamina dura-like border, and it is often surrounded by a radiolucent capsule. Clinically, the patient is asymptomatic, but presents with one or more bony hard nodular, pedunculated or flat protuberances on the surface of the maxilla and/or the mandible. A synonym is the *osteoma*.

Fibrosarcoma

A *fibrosarcoma* is a malignant fibroblastic tumor that is characterized by varying amounts of collagen formation and the absence of bone production. Typically, it is a single lesion showing a predilection for the long bones, with only rare cases located in either the maxilla or the mandible. However, within the jaws, there is a predilection for the posterior regions (e.g. molar–ramus) of the mandible. The average patient is between 20 and 40 years of age at the time of diagnosis, but a fibrosarcoma may occur at any age and there is no sexual or racial predilection. A fibrosarcoma often appears as an irregular radiolucent lesion with ill-defined borders. It is an aggressive, fast-growing lesion that causes diffuse bone destruction, often in less than 6 months. As the lesion does not have any distinct borders, it consequently blends into the surrounding bone. Within the radiolucent lesion, there are often nodular or diffuse calcifications that represent remnants of bone that the fibrosarcoma did not fully destroy. This is indicative of the rapidity with which the tumor spreads throughout the bone. There is also a characteristic thinning and perforation of the cortical plate. Once the fibrosarcoma pervades the cortical plate, the cortical plate resembles a grate or a mesh because of the numerous perforations through it. It is notable that a *sunburst* appearance is not produced as in an osteosarcoma. Clinically, the patient often presents with pain, swelling, loosening of the teeth, paresthesia and hyperplastic gingiva.

Fibrous dysplasia

Fibrous dysplasia is a slow-growing, benign, fibro-osseous lesion of unknown etiology, characterized by the formation of fibrous connective tissue within the affected bone(s). Various theories concerning the pathogenesis, such as trauma or congenital development, have been proposed, but a unanimous consensus still does not exist. This lesion is classified into three categories: monostotic fibrous dysplasia, polyostotic fibrous dysplasia and Albright's syndrome. *Monostotic fibrous dysplasia* characteristically affects only a portion of a single bone. *Polyostotic fibrous dysplasia* affects more than one bone and is associated with *café-au-lait spots* ☢. *Albright's syndrome* is characterized by polyostotic bone involvement, *café-au-lait spots* and endocrine involvement (e.g. precocious puberty). All three classifications may affect any bone. Within the maxilla and the mandible, fibrous dysplasia is predominantly found in the posterior regions of the maxilla and less frequently it is located in the posterior regions of the mandible. The size of the lesion is quite variable, ranging from 1 cm to total involvement of the bone(s). There is a predilection for females under 30 years of age, but it can occur in either sex, in any age group and develop in all races. Fibrous dysplasia is quite variable. Initially, it appears as a small, unilocular or multilocular radiolucency with well-defined borders (Figs X1 and X2). The lesion develops into an ill-defined radiolucent area (i.e. lacking a radiopaque rim), with zones of sclerotic bone within it. This stage is often described as having a mottled appearance. The late stage is characterized by thinning and expansion of the cortical plate and an increasing amount of sclerotic bone within the lesion, giving it a *ground glass appearance* ☢ (Fig. X3). It is important to note that outside of the lesion, there are not any sclerotic changes occurring within the bone. Also, the lamina dura is destroyed when the lesion involves a tooth. Clinically, the patient often presents

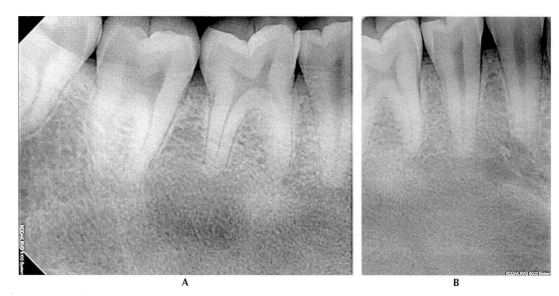

A   B

Fig. X3 Ground glass appearance. (Source: Shumway BS, Foster TS (2011) Pathology of the jaw: the importance of radiographs. *J Can Dent Assoc* 77: b132. Reproduced with permission of the Canadian Dental Association.)

with a painless swelling, while less frequently nasal obstruction and tooth displacement may be observed. Synonyms include *osteitic fibrosa, osteofibroma, localized osteodystrophia* and *Jaffe's type fibrous dysplasia.*

Foreign body

Any substance introduced into an individual either voluntarily or involuntarily must be properly interpreted by the clinician. Involuntary inclusion refers to *iatrogenic* causes related to a medical or dental procedure (e.g. broken instrument) or during an unrelated accident (e.g. gunshot wound, auto incident). The shape, size, location, density and number of foreign bodies are variable. Dental artifacts may include restorative materials, cements, broken endodontic files, broken surgical burs, etc. In addition, radiopacities located in edentulous areas on x-ray images may have been introduced into the socket during a dental extraction procedure (e.g. remnant of an occlusal restoration). A thorough review of a patient's clinical history will often reveal the source of the foreign material.

Giant cell granuloma, central

A *giant cell granuloma* is a term that was first used in the 1950s to describe and to categorize giant cell tumors of the maxilla and mandible. Controversy still exists as to whether the giant cell tumor of bone and the central giant cell granuloma are actually separate entities. The central giant cell granuloma is a slow-growing lesion rarely found outside of the maxilla and mandible. Typically, the anterior region of the mandible is affected and less frequently the anterior region of the maxilla. The lesion will average from 1 to 3 cm in diameter, but it could involve the entire bone. The central giant cell granuloma is rarely found in individuals over 21 years of age and females are most often affected with this lesion. The patient's past medical and dental history frequently indicates prior trauma to the area. Typically it appears as a single, multiloculated radiolucency, having a *soap bubble* appearance (Fig. X1) with smooth, well-defined margins. Often thinning, expansion and perforation of the cortical plate ensue. However it may appear as a unilocular radiolucency and the margins may be ragged. The patient often presents with a painless swelling and displaced teeth. Pain and root resorption occur less frequently. The giant cell granuloma is a self-limiting lesion that occasionally subsides spontaneously and seldom recurs.

Giant cell tumor

A *giant cell tumor* is a benign, yet aggressive, lesion, classically located within the long bones, particularly about the knee. Few cases have been located within the maxilla and mandible. The mandible is more frequently involved than the maxilla, with both showing a predilection for the anterior region. Typically, the giant cell tumor is a single lesion, averaging from 1 to 3 cm in diameter. The average patient is between 21 and 40 years of age at the time of diagnosis, but the tumor may be found in any age group. There is a slight predilection for occurrence in females. Because the lesion is slow growing, it may be years before the patient is cognizant of any unusual symptoms. Radiologically, the giant cell tumor is quite variable. Frequently, the tumor appears as a multiloculated radiolucency with smooth, well-defined borders and with thinning and expansion of the cortical plate (Fig. X1). However, the giant cell tumor may perforate the cortical plate. The patient often complains of pain, swelling, paresthesia and loosening of the teeth. Inadequate enucleation of the tumor often results in recurrence of the lesion. Synonyms include *chronic hemorrhagic osteomyelitis, osteoclastoma, myeloid sarcoma* and *giant cell sarcoma*.

Granuloma, periapical

A *periapical granuloma* is a localized mass of chronic granulation tissue formed in response to pulpal infection. Any tooth in either the maxilla or the mandible may be affected. It may either be single or multiple in number and the size of the lesion may vary from a few millimeters to over a centimeter in diameter. The periapical

granuloma has reportedly occurred in all age groups, but it is most frequently found in patients aged 20–30 years. It has generally been accepted that there is no sexual or racial predilection. The periapical granuloma appears as a round or oval-shaped radiolucency and it may or may not have well-defined borders. Also, there is a partial loss of the lamina dura in the affected region. A patient's past dental history will often indicate a record of pulpitis as a result of caries or, less frequently, an incident of trauma to the affected tooth. Typically, the duration of time between the pulpitis or the trauma to the tooth and the diagnosis of the periapical granuloma is less than 1 year. Histologic examination is necessary to differentiate the granuloma from a cyst or an abscess. Clinically, the patient often is asymptomatic. However, if the etiology is caries, then the patient may experience discomfort from percussion and chewing. The affected tooth is non-vital and it may appear darker in color than the surrounding normal teeth. Synonyms include *apical granuloma* and *periapical rarefying osteitis*.

Hemangioma

A *hemangioma* of bone is a benign neoplasm characterized by a proliferation of blood vessels. Typically, the hemangioma is a single lesion, but it can be multiple in numbers. The average patient is between 10 and 30 years of age at the time of diagnosis but it may occur in patients of all ages. There does not appear to be any racial or sexual predilection present. The etiology of a hemangioma remains uncertain, but often there is a history of other vascular disorders or tooth extraction in the affected area. It is a slow-growing lesion with duration of time varying from weeks to years. The hemangioma is predominantly located in the spinal vertebrae. Less frequently, it is found in the posterior regions of the maxilla and the mandible, particularly in the mandible. The size of the lesion is quite variable ranging from 1 cm to total involvement of

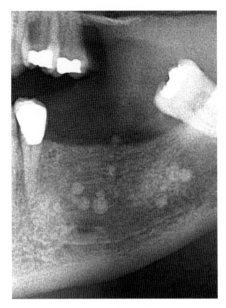

Fig. X4 Phleboliths.

the bone(s). The hemangioma is quite variable in appearance. It ranges from a well-defined multilocular radiolucency with well-defined margins having a *soap bubble* appearance (Fig. X1) to a diffuse, oval or round unilocular radiolucency with irregular, indistinct margins. Occasionally the hemangioma has been reported to have a *sunray* appearance inside the radiolucency as a result of bone proliferation from within the lesion. On average, the hemangioma is 1–2 cm in diameter. In addition, there frequently is erosion of the lamina dura, root resorption and phleboliths (Fig. X4) within the lesion. Clinically, the hemangioma presents as a painless swelling, with loosening of the teeth and bleeding around the necks of the teeth.

Hyperparathyroidism

Hyperparathyroidism is a metabolic bone disease resulting from an increased secretion of parathyroid hormone. This increased hormone secretion results in a generalized decrease in image density of the skeletal bones including the maxilla and mandible, giving them a *ground glass* appearance. Also, hyperparathyroidism leads to the partial or total loss of the lamina dura around all of the teeth and a fading or a disappearance of the radiopaque lines bordering the maxillary sinus and the nasal cavity. In association with it, there are often brown tumors, which are vascular intraosseous soft tissue masses. The brown tumor appears as a well-circumscribed radiolucent area identical to the giant cell granuloma and it is most often observed in the mandible, clavicle, ribs and pelvis. Females over 30 years of age are most often affected, but there is no racial predilection. Clinically, the patient presents with loosening of the teeth, nausea, a history of bone fractures, hypercalcemia and hypophosphatemia. It is notable that after treatment of hyperparathyroidism, the healed bone is often very dense and never appears quite normal. A synonym is *osteitis fibrosa*.

Metastatic tumor

A characteristic of malignant tumors is their ability to metastasize at some stage of development to sites distant from their origin. Metastatic tumors to the maxilla and/or the mandible are quite rare. However, the paucity of cases reported in the literature indicates that the most prevalent metastatic sites of origin are the breast, lung, kidney and prostate gland. Typically, the posterior regions of the mandible are affected. Should the condyle be involved, almost a definitive diagnosis of a metastatic tumor is possible, as a result of the rarity of lesions that affect it. The average patient is over 50 years of age at the time of the diagnosis and there is no apparent sexual or racial predilection. There are not any characteristic clinical or radiologic findings associated with a metastatic tumor. It may be single or multiple in number, range from one to several centimeters in size, appear unilocular or multilocular, have well-defined or ill-defined borders, be regular or irregular in outline and can be radiolucent or radiopaque in density. Typically, however, it appears as an ill-defined radiolucent lesion. The patient may present with pain, swelling, paresthesia, trismus, mobile teeth and a poor healing tooth socket from an earlier extraction. It may also present as a single extruded tooth in an otherwise normal appearing dentition.

Multiple myeloma

Multiple myeloma is a malignant tumor of plasma cells, primarily characterized by widespread bone destruction. Typically, it is found in patients over 60 years of age, rarely being found in anyone below 50 years of age. There is a predilection for black males. Bones containing hematopoietic marrow such as the vertebrae, ribs, pelvis and skull are most frequently affected. When the bones of the oral cavity are involved, it predominantly occurs in the posterior regions of the mandible. Compared to histiocytosis-X, the size of a myelomatous lesion is quite small, averaging from 1 to 2 cm in diameter. Also, there are greater numbers of lesions (unless the lesions coalesce) present in the individual with multiple myeloma than in patients with histiocytosis-X. On rare occasions, the myeloma has been reported to occur as a single lesion, but controversy exists as to whether it is a separate entity or simply an early developmental stage of the multiple myeloma. Classically, multiple myelomas appear as *punched-out* ☢ radiolucent areas of bone destruction which do not show trabeculae within them, nor any sclerotic zones around their periphery. Within the mandible, there is often expansion, thinning and perforation of the cortical plate. The patient's past medical and/or dental history often indicates anemia, renal dysfunction, weight loss, a history of multiple bone fractures and numerous extractions of loose teeth. Clinically, the patient often presents with pain, swelling, weakness and mobile teeth.

Synonyms include *plasma cell myeloma, plasmacytic myeloma* and *myelomatosis*.

Myxoma

Myxoma is a benign odontogenic tumor that is believed to originate from the mesenchymal portion of the tooth germ. The tumor is very rarely located outside of the maxilla and the mandible. It shows a slight predilection for the mandible over the maxilla, with the posterior regions primarily being affected. The average patient is between 10 and 50 years of age, but reports exist of the tumor occurring in patients of all ages. Past dental histories often reveal the occurrence of congenitally absent or unerupted teeth. However, there does not appear to be any racial or sexual predilection. The myxoma is quite variable in appearance, ranging from a single, multiloculated radiolucent lesion with well-defined borders having a *honeycomb appearance* ☢ (Fig. X5) to a unilocular, cyst-like radiolucency with ill-defined borders. The margins often appear scalloped and there frequently is bony destruction of the cortical plate. Occasionally, there may be root resorption. The size of the lesion is also quite variable, ranging from 1 to 10 cm in diameter. Clinically, the patient presents with a painless swelling and possibly loosened or displaced teeth. The myxoma has also been found to recur frequently. Synonyms include *odontogenic myxoma, myxofibroma* and *odontogenic fibromyxoma*.

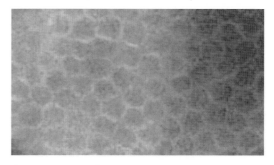

Fig. X5 Honeycomb appearance.

Odontoma, complex

See Section W.

Odontoma, compound

See Section W.

Osseous dysplasia

Osseous dysplasia is a benign fibro-osseous lesion of unknown etiology. Typically, it is asymptomatic and as a result it is often found incidentally on intraoral x-ray images during routine examinations. Three clinical presentations of osseous dysplasia exist: periapical osseous dysplasia, focal osseous dysplasia and florid osseous dysplasia. *Periapical and focal osseous dysplasia* share the same clinical, radiologic and histologic features, only differing on the basis of location. Periapical osseous dysplasia is typically diffusely located in the mandibular incisor region, while focal osseous dysplasia is typically a well-defined lesion located in the posterior region of the mandible. Because periapical osseous dysplasia frequently is associated with the apices of several teeth, it may be misdiagnosed as being multiple lesions. The location of *florid osseous dysplasia* is more generalized and it is found in at least two quadrants. Osseous dysplasia is quite variable and can be classified into early, mixed and late stages of development. The early stage is characterized as a small periapical radiolucent defect. Note that if multiple neighboring teeth are involved, then a fusion of these radiolucencies may give rise to a single, large, less clearly defined radiolucent lesion. The mixed stage is characterized by the formation of minute radiopacities within the radiolucent lesion. The late stage is characterized by the coalescing of the calcified structures within the radiolucent area, resulting in a dense radiopacity. The average size of a lesion is 1–2 cm in diameter. Florid osseous dysplasia appears as multiple, irregularly-shaped radiopacities surrounded by thin, radiolucent borders located in multiple quadrants. Osseous dysplasia shows a predilection for middle-aged black females. Clinical examination will reveal that the involved tooth or teeth are vital. Osseous dysplasia is self-limiting and typically does not require treatment. Clinical and radiologic follow-up is recommended. Synonyms include *cemento-osseous dysplasia, cementoma, true attached cementoma, periapical cemental dysplasia, sclerosing cementum, periapical fibrous dysplasia* and *periapical fibro-osteoma*.

Ossifying fibroma

An *ossifying fibroma* is a central fibro-osseous lesion. It is a single lesion located predominantly in the posterior regions of the mandible and, less frequently, in the anterior regions of the maxilla. The lesion develops close to the roots of teeth and often results in tooth displacement. Typically, the average patient is aged 20–40 years at the time of the diagnosis, but the tumor may be found in any age group. It is notable that there is a slight predilection for females. While the etiology remains unknown, there is often a history of trauma to the affected area. Radiologically, the cementifying–ossifying fibroma is quite variable. Initially, it may appear as a unilocular or multilocular radiolucency with well-defined borders. During the intermediary stage, it is transformed into a mixed radiolucent–radiopaque lesion having a *ground glass* or a *cotton wool appearance* ☢ (Figs X3 and X6). The late stage of the tumor is characterized by a well-circumscribed radiopaque lesion surrounded by a uniform radiolucent rim. In addition, there may be expansion of the cortical plate. Clinically, the ossifying fibroma is a slow-growing, painless lesion. As a result, the patient is often not cognizant of any unusual symptoms for years. Synonyms include *cementifying fibroma, ossifying fibroma, osteofibroma, fibrous osteoma, fibro-osseous lesion of bone* and *benign non-odontogenic tumor of the jaw.*

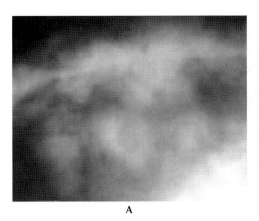
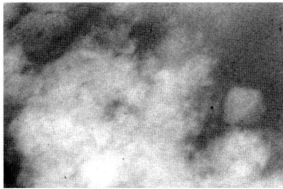

A   B

Fig. X6 Cotton wool appearance.

Osteomyelitis

Osteomyelitis is an inflammation of bone commonly initiated by either an abscessed tooth or the result of a post-surgical infection. There are many different forms of osteomyelitis. However, they can be categorized into acute and chronic phases. Occasionally the source of infection may not be known. Inflammation can involve all of the bony components: cortical and cancellous bone and the periosteum. The mandible is more commonly affected than the maxilla because of its comparatively poorer blood supply, although either may be affected. CBCT imaging is the modality of choice. Acute osteomyelitis occurs in all age groups, with males being affected more commonly. It often has a rapid onset, with pain, swelling and a purulent discharge in the affected area. Teeth in the affected area may be mobile and sensitive to percussion. In the early stage of acute osteomyelitis there may not be any changes seen radiologically. Gradually, however, there will be a decrease in bone density that may be isolated locally or widespread. Additionally, there may be the appearance of sclerotic patches and the formation of bone sequestrae. Should the acute phase of osteomyelitis be inadequately resolved, a chronic diffuse sclerosing form of osteomyelitis may develop. Chronic osteomyelitis predominantly occurs in the posterior aspect of the mandible and is associated with an increase in bone deposition. Gradually the appearance will change from a mixed radiolucent–radiopaque area to a dense radiopacity. Patient's signs and symptoms may include recurring episodes of swelling, pain, fever and lymphadenopathy. Synonyms for osteomyelitis include *acute suppurative osteomyelitis, pyogenic osteomyelitis, subacute suppurative osteomyelitis, Garre's osteomyelitis, proliferative osteomyelitis, periostitis ossificans, chronic osteomyelitis, chronic diffuse suppurative osteomyelitis, chronic non-suppurative osteomyelitis, chronic osteomyelitis proliferative osteomyelitis* and *Garre's non-suppurative osteomyelitis.*

Osteopetrosis

Osteopetrosis is a disease of unknown etiology characterized by a generalized thickening and *sclerosis of bone* ☢. Two forms of osteopetrosis exist. *Osteopetrosis congenita* is a malignant form, commonly seen in infants or young children and it is typically fatal as a result of anemia, massive hemorrhage or rampant bone infection. *Osteopetrosis tarda* is a benign form and it may be diagnosed during childhood or during any stage of adult life. This latter type may be asymptomatic and the patient's lifespan does not seem to be shortened. There is no sexual or racial predilection in either form. Both forms show an increase in the density and thickness of the bones of the entire skeleton. As a result, the bones have a homogeneous, symmetrically sclerotic appearance. The cortex and the medullary cavity of each of the bones become indistinguishable. There is loss of the lamina dura and, in severe cases, the paranasal sinuses become opacified. Clinically, during the early stages of the disease, the patient may be asymptomatic and consequently osteopetrosis may be diagnosed inadvertently during routine radiologic examination. However, during the later stages of the disease, the patient often presents with a thickening of the skull, deafness, blindness, facial paralysis, poor healing capabilities, a history of repeated fractures and anemia. Synonyms include *Albers–Schonberg disease*, *marble bone disease* and *osteosclerosis fragilis generalsata*.

Osteoporosis

Osteoporosis is a common bone disease in which the density of bone is diminished. There are no symptoms in the early stages. Patients are often unaware of their condition until a fracture occurs. Ostoeporosis of the maxilla and mandible will appear as a generalized rarefaction. Generalized thinning of the cortical plates and thinning or loss of trabeculae will be evident. It is more commonly found in post-menopausal white and Asian females. Risk factors include small stature, taking medications (e.g. for treatment of lupus, asthma, thyroid deficiencies and prostate cancer), low calcium intake, inactive lifestyle, smoking and drinking excessive alcohol. With increasing age, both women and men frequently will suffer a fracture of a hip, wrist or vertebra as a result of osteoporosis. Antiresorptive mediations such as *bisphosphonates* ☢ are commonly used to treat post-menopausal osteoporosis.

Bisphosphonates have been associated with unusual fractures in the femur.

Osteosarcoma

Osteosarcoma is a malignant neoplasm in which the tumor cells produce immature bone. Typically, it involves one or more bones, showing a predilection for occurrence in the long bones and the knee, with fewer than 10% of the cases reported in the maxilla or mandible. The average patient is aged 30–40 years at the time of diagnosis. Cases involving the maxilla and/or the mandible often develop in patients who are 10 years older than those individuals with tumors found in the long bones. There is no racial predilection, but males are more frequently affected. While the etiology remains unknown, there often is a history of trauma to the area. It is a fast-growing, aggressive lesion with a duration varying from weeks to years. The mandible is involved approximately twice as often as the maxilla and it predominantly occurs in the anterior region of either bone. The osteosarcoma can be classified into early (osteolytic), intermediate (osteolytic and osteoblastic) and late (sclerotic) stages. The early stage is characterized by a generalized widening of the periodontal ligament spaces and an ill-defined pear- or oval-shaped radiolucency. The intermediate stage reveals a concurrent process of resorption and deposition of bone, giving rise to an ill-defined mixed radiolucent–radiopaque region. The late stage is characterized by a dense radiopaque lesion, often displaying the classic *sunburst* or *sun-ray* appearance (Fig. X7), with or without the partial destruction of the cortical plate. The size of the lesion is quite variable, ranging from one to several centimeters in diameter. Clinically, the symptoms include pain, malocclusion, swelling, paresthesia and loosening of the teeth; also, the osteosarcoma is often associated with Paget's disease. A synonym is *osteogenic sarcoma*.

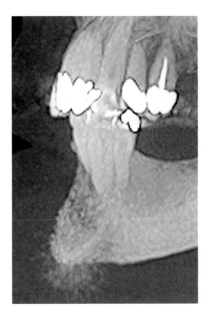

Fig. X7 Sunburst appearance.

Paget's disease

Paget's disease is a disease of unknown etiology that is characterized by concurrent destruction and formation of bone. This condition appears on average in patients over 40 years of age and it rarely appears in patients younger than 30 years of age. There is a predilection for occurrence in males (the male : female ratio being approximately 2 : 1), and approximately 50% of the cases demonstrate a hereditary pattern. Patients are not cognizant of any unusual symptoms until the disease is of several years' duration. However, in the later stages, patients often complain of pain, deafness, visual loss, ill-fitting dentures and hats that have become too small. Typically, Paget's disease involves more than one bone, mainly affecting the bones of the lower extremities, the neck and the skull. This often results in a bowing of the lower extremities, scoliosis, kyphosis and an enlargement of the affected bone. Paget's disease is also associated with osteosarcoma. The size of the lesion is quite variable, ranging from a few centimeters to total involvement of the affected

bone(s). Its appearance can be classified into the early (osteolytic), intermediate (mixed) and late (osteoblastic) stages. The early stage is characterized by radiolucencies of variable size, often becoming confluent with sharp, somewhat jagged contours and also potentially having a *ground glass* appearance. The intermediate stage reflects the concurrent process of resorption and deposition of bone. This results in an ill-defined lesion with widening of the cortex, enlargement of the bone and a *cotton wool* appearance (Fig. X6). The late stage is characterized by a coalescing of the radiopacities, resulting in dense, irregular areas of calcification, a loss of the lamina dura and frequent bone fractures. A synonym is *osteitis deformans*.

Phlebolith, intraoral

Intraoral *phleboliths* are calcified thrombi found within the soft tissues. They are characteristically associated with cases of cavernous hemangiomas. Consequently, phleboliths appear predominantly in individuals under 30 years of age, but they may arise in any age group. There is no racial or sexual predilection. Phleboliths typically appear as multiple, small, rounded radiopacities having concentric structures, with radiolucent centers (Fig. X4). The average size of each phlebolith is from 1 to 3 mm in diameter. Sometimes, they are referred to as having a buckshot appearance. Clinically, the patient often presents with a painless swelling. It is notable that this swelling is not affected by eating, as with sialoliths. Phleboliths are frequently associated with hemangiomas.

Rhinolith

A rhinolith is a mass that arises from the deposition of calcific salts around the nuclei of blood, mucous or foreign bodies. The rhinolith is specifically located within the nasal fossa. A rhinolith may be single or multiple in number and it may vary from a few millimeters to a few centimeters in size. It is most commonly found in individuals younger than 40 years of age, but it may occur in any age group. Also, there is no sexual or racial predilection. A rhinolith appears as a regular or irregular radiopacity with well-defined margins. The patient's past medical and dental histories often reveal an incident of an earlier traumatic extraction or an instance during childhood when a small object (e.g. cherry pit) was inserted into the patient's nose. A rhinolith is a slow-growing mass and the individual may not be cognizant of any unusual symptoms for years. Some patients may complain of headaches, nasal obstruction and/or discharge, laryngitis or epistaxis, while other individuals may be totally asymptomatic. A synonym for a rhinolith is *nasal calculus*.

Salivary gland tumors, benign and malignant

Benign and malignant tumors of the salivary glands rarely manifest themselves in the jaws. Typically, both types of tumors present as single lesions occurring predominantly in the posterior aspects of either the maxilla and/or the mandible. There is no sexual or racial predilection; however the benign and malignant salivary gland tumors typically occur in individuals more than 30 years of age. Malignant tumors are particularly prevalent in the older age categories. It is notable that while a benign tumor has a duration varying from months to years prior to its diagnosis, a malignant lesion generally only has a duration of weeks to months prior to its diagnosis. The benign salivary gland tumor usually appears as a well-defined, round or oval-shaped radiolucent lesion having a radiopaque periphery. The malignant salivary gland tumor often appears as an ill-defined, irregular-shaped radiolucency that lacks a radiopaque periphery. The size of both of the lesions averages from 1 to 5 cm in diameter. Clinically, the benign salivary gland tumor presents as a painless swelling, while the malignant salivary

gland tumor may present with or without pain and/or swelling. Synonyms for benign salivary gland tumors include *benign adenoma* and *adenoma*, while a synonym for a malignant salivary gland tumor is *adenocarcinoma*.

Scar, periapical

A *periapical scar* is a well-defined or an ill-defined radiolucent lesion found at the apex of a tooth that has a history of periapical involvement and endodontic treatment. It represents an area where the healing process terminated in the formation of collagen rather than bone. The size of the periapical scar is variable, ranging from less than 1 cm to several centimeters in diameter. It may be located in any of the tooth-bearing areas of the maxilla and mandible. There is no sexual or racial predilection and it may be found in any age group. Clinically the tooth is asymptomatic and the periapical scar is often incidentally discovered during routine intraoral imaging. A synonym is *apical scar*.

Sialolith

Sialoliths are calcareous concretions that slowly develop within a salivary duct or a salivary gland. They form by the deposition of calcium salts around a central nidus, which may be a foreign body, desquamated epithelial cells or bacteria. Sialoliths may be single or multiple in number, and they may vary from less than 1 cm to over 12 cm in size. They are most commonly found in middle-aged adults, but they occur in all age groups. There is no sexual or racial predilection. The submandibular gland and duct are most frequently involved with sialolithiasis, followed by the parotid gland and duct and the sublingual gland and duct. On extremely rare occasions, sialoliths have involved the minor salivary glands and ducts. The sialolith usually appears as a round or oval, uniformly dense radiopacity, with either regular or irregular margins (see Fig. Y15). Clinically, the patient often complains of a painful swelling, particularly during eating. It is also notable that the sialoliths are not attached to any bones. Synonyms include *salivary duct calculus*, *salivary duct stone* and *salivary calculi*.

Torus

A *torus* is a slow-growing bony excrescence of unknown etiology that may be found either singly or multiple in number. It is either located on the lateral aspect of the lingual surface of the mandible, particularly in the premolar–molar region, and is referred to as a *torus mandibularis* or it is located in the midline of the palate and is referred to as a *torus palatinus*. The shape and size of any torus is quite variable. It may appear flat, lobular or oval and it may range from a few millimeters to several centimeters in length (see Figs M25 and U18). There is no sexual predilection. The average patient is under 30 years of age when the lesion is first diagnosed and it stops increasing in size by middle-age. A torus appears as an oval-shaped radiopacity, usually with well-defined borders. Clinically, the lesion is asymptomatic.

Y Lagniappe ☢ (Miscellaneous Oddities)

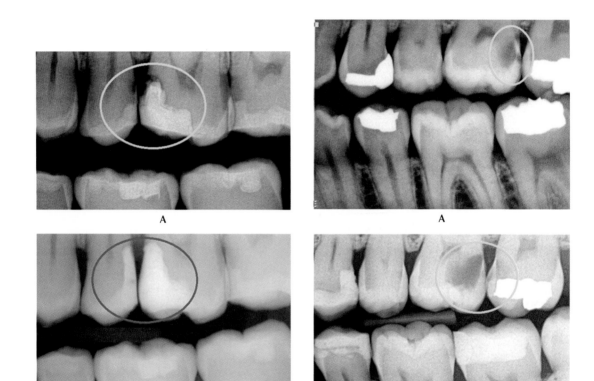

Fig. Y1 A. Poorly filled interproximal composite restorations on distal of no. 13 and mesial no. 14. B. Re-treated nos 13 and 14 with good composite restorations. Note that recurrent decay was not the cause of the radiolucency in this instance.

Fig. Y2 A. Carious lesion in distal no.14. B. Progression of the untreated carious lesion 6 years later.

Fundamentals of Oral and Maxillofacial Radiology, First Edition. J. Sean Hubar.
© 2017 John Wiley & Sons, Inc. Published 2017 by John Wiley & Sons, Inc.
Companion website: www.wiley.com/go/hubar/radiology

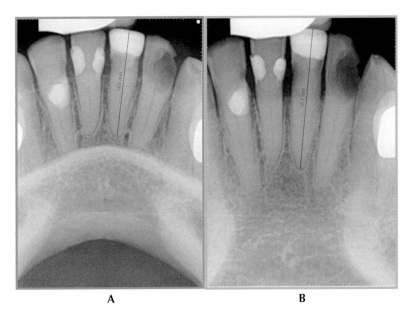

Fig. Y3 Measurements of a tooth imaged twice (consecutively) with altered vertical angulation. The results show significant differences in tooth measurements. Conclusion: measurements taken on conventional images often are inaccurate because software measuring tools cannot compensate for image distortion (e.g. elongation or foreshortening).

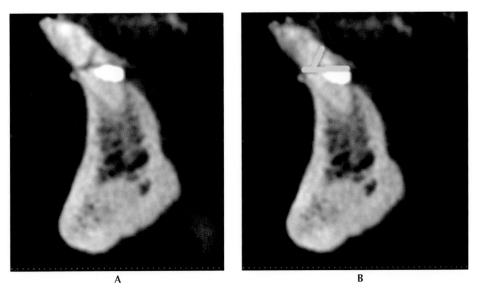

Fig. Y4 Misdirected anchoring device for sleep apnea device resulting in root fractures (highlighted in B). The anchoring device was intended to be inserted into bone inferior to the root.

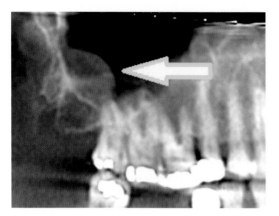

Fig. Y5 Mucosal antral cyst: dome-shaped radiopacity. Do not confuse this with a sinus lift procedure as shown in Fig. Y14.

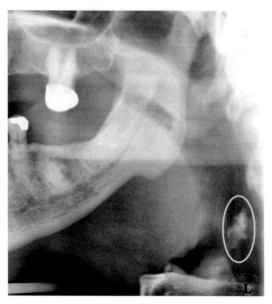

Fig. Y6 Carotid artery calcification: irregular-shaped radiopacity.

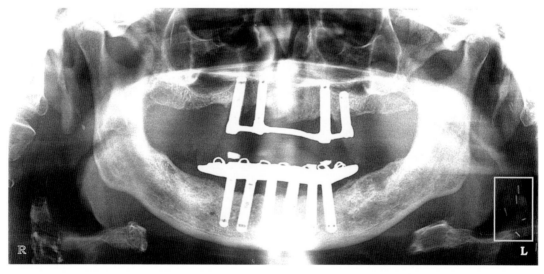

Fig. Y7 Internal radiotherapy involves surgically implanting tiny pellets or rods (multiple small radiopacities) containing radioactive materials in or near a tumor.

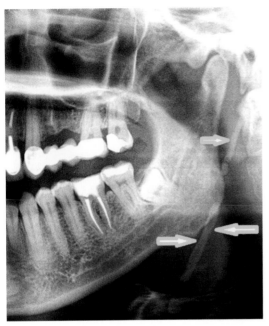

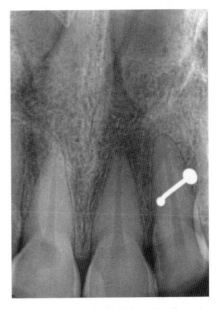

Fig. Y10 Nose piercing: barbell-shaped radiopacity.

Fig. Y8 Calcification of the stylohyoid ligament: elongated, segmented radiopacity.

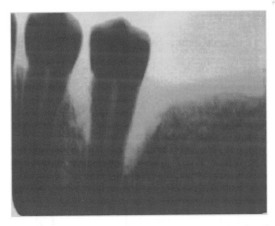

Fig. Y9 Colorized x-ray image highlighting localized angular periodontal bone loss.

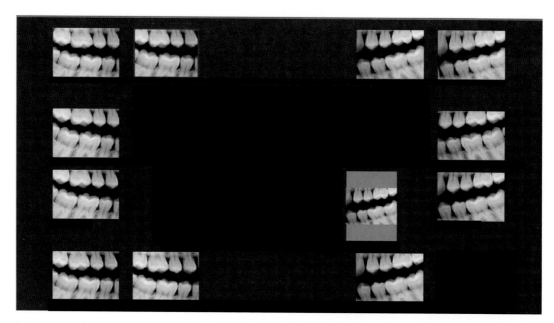

Fig. Y11 Example of multiple exposures taken in the hope of obtaining one perfect image. Biologic effects of radiation are cumulative. Follow the ALADA principle.

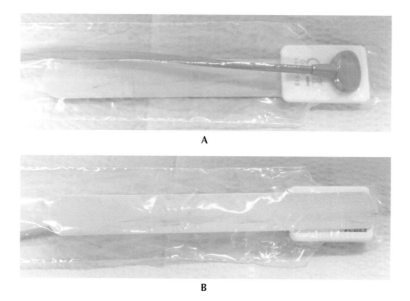

A

B

Fig. Y12 Tongue depressor.

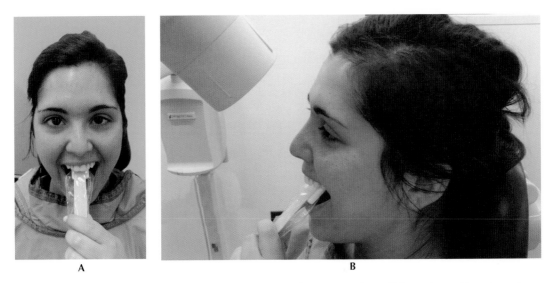

Fig. Y13 Patient holding the receptor in position. A tongue depressor works well beneath a rubber dam when a conventional receptor holder may not work.

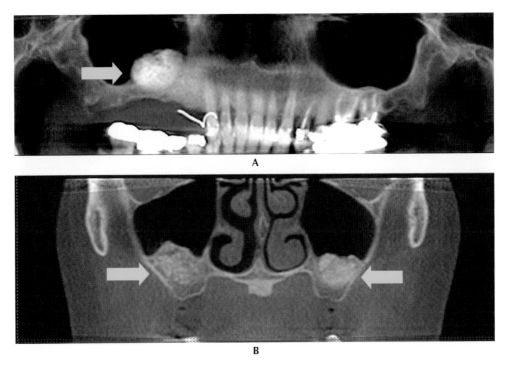

Fig. Y14 Post-sinus lift surgery: radiopaque mass in the maxillary right sinus (arrows). A. CBCT panoramic view. B. CBCT coronal view. This radiopacity should not be misinterpreted as sinusitis.

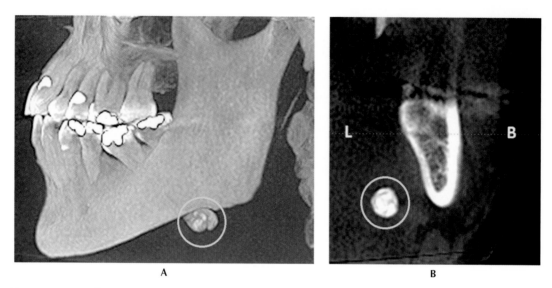

Fig. Y15 A. Sagittal view of a sialolith. B. Coronal view of a sialolith, showing it located on the lingual aspect of the mandible.

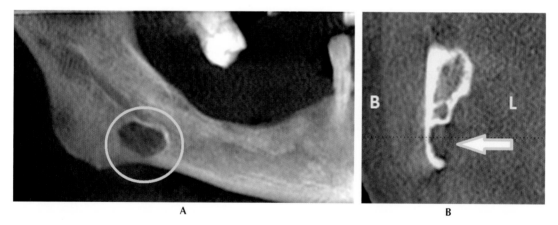

Fig. Y16 A. Sagittal view of a Stafne bone cyst. B. Coronal view revealing the radiolucent concavity attributed to the Stafne bone cyst.

Part Three   Appendices

Appendix 1
FDA Recommendations for Prescribing Dental X-ray Images

Fundamentals of Oral and Maxillofacial Radiology, First Edition. J. Sean Hubar.
© 2017 John Wiley & Sons, Inc. Published 2017 by John Wiley & Sons, Inc.
Companion website: www.wiley.com/go/hubar/radiology

RECOMMENDATIONS FOR PRESCRIBING DENTAL RADIOGRAPHS

These recommendations are subject to clinical judgment and may not apply to every patient. They are to be used by dentists only after reviewing the patient's health history and completing a clinical examination. Even though radiation exposure from dental radiographs is low, once a decision to obtain radiographs is made it is the dentist's responsibility to follow the ALARA Principle (As Low as Reasonably Achievable) to minimize the patient's exposure.

TYPE OF ENCOUNTER	PATIENT AGE AND DENTAL DEVELOPMENTAL STAGE				
	Child with Primary Dentition (prior to eruption of first permanent tooth)	Child with Transitional Dentition (after eruption of first permanent tooth)	Adolescent with Permanent Dentition (prior to eruption of third molars)	Adult, Dentate or Partially Edentulous	Adult, Edentulous
New Patient* being evaluated for oral diseases	Individualized radiographic exam consisting of selected periapical/occlusal views and/or posterior bitewings if proximal surfaces cannot be visualized or probed. Patients without evidence of disease and with open proximal contacts may not require a radiographic exam at this time.	Individualized radiographic exam consisting of posterior bitewings with panoramic exam or posterior bitewings and selected periapical images.		Individualized radiographic exam consisting of posterior bitewings with panoramic exam or posterior bitewings. A full mouth intraoral radiographic exam is preferred when the patient has clinical evidence of generalized oral disease or a history of extensive dental treatment.	Individualized radiographic exam, based on clinical signs and symptoms.
Recall Patient* with clinical caries or at increased risk for caries**	Posterior bitewing exam at 6-12 month intervals if proximal surfaces cannot be examined visually or with a probe		Posterior bitewing exam at 6-18 month intervals		Not applicable
Recall Patient* with no clinical caries and not at increased risk for caries**	Posterior bitewing exam at 12-24 month intervals if proximal surfaces cannot be examined visually or with a probe		Posterior bitewing exam at 18-36 month intervals	Posterior bitewing exam at 24-36 month intervals	Not applicable
Recall Patient* with periodontal disease	Clinical judgment as to the need for and type of radiographic images for the evaluation of periodontal disease. Imaging may consist of, but is not limited to, selected bitewing and/or periapical images of areas where periodontal disease (other than nonspecific gingivitis) can be demonstrated clinically.				Not applicable
Patient (New and Recall) for monitoring of dentofacial growth and development, and/or assessment of dental/skeletal relationships	Clinical judgment as to the need for and type of radiographic images for evaluation and/or monitoring of dentofacial growth and development or assessment of dental and skeletal relationships		Clinical judgment as to need for and type of radiographic images for evaluation and/or monitoring of dentofacial growth and development. Panoramic or periapical exam to assess developing third molars	Usually not indicated for monitoring of growth and development. Clinical judgment as to the need for and type of radiographic image for evaluation of dental and skeletal relationships.	
Patient with other circumstances including, but not limited to, proposed or existing implants, other dental and craniofacial pathoses, restorative/endodontic needs, treated periodontal disease and caries remineralization	Clinical judgment as to need for and type of radiographic images for evaluation and/or monitoring of these conditions				

RECOMMENDATIONS FOR PRESCRIBING DENTAL RADIOGRAPHS

*Clinical situations for which radiographs may be indicated include, but are not limited to:

A. Positive Historical Findings

1. Previous periodontal or endodontic treatment
2. History of pain or trauma
3. Familial history of dental anomalies
4. Postoperative evaluation of healing
5. Remineralization monitoring
6. Presence of implants, previous implant-related pathosis or evaluation for implant placement

B. Positive Clinical Signs/Symptoms

1. Clinical evidence of periodontal disease
2. Large or deep restorations
3. Deep carious lesions
4. Malposed or clinically impacted teeth
5. Swelling
6. Evidence of dental/facial trauma
7. Mobility of teeth
8. Sinus tract ("fistula")
9. Clinically suspected sinus pathosis
10. Growth abnormalities
11. Oral involvement in known or suspected systemic disease
12. Positive neurologic findings in the head and neck
13. Evidence of foreign objects
14. Pain and/or dysfunction of the temporomandibular joint
15. Facial asymmetry
16. Abutment teeth for fixed or removable partial prosthesis
17. Unexplained bleeding
18. Unexplained sensitivity of teeth
19. Unusual eruption, spacing or migration of teeth
20. Unusual tooth morphology, calcification or color
21. Unexplained absence of teeth
22. Clinical tooth erosion
23. Peri-implantitis

**Factors increasing risk for caries may be assessed using the ADA Caries Risk Assessment forms (0 – 6 years of age and over 6 years of age).

Appendix 2
X-radiation Concerns of Patients: Question and Answer Format

Patients may read an article in a magazine or on the internet, hear a report in the news or listen to other so-called authorities with information that contradicts the x-ray imaging protocol practiced by their personal dentists. A patient may then confront their dental professional about these concerns. The typical patient wants a concise answer that is easy to understand. In cases where the need or frequency of x-ray exposure is questioned, dental auxiliaries are often the dental professional of choice for the answers. This author believes that the public's perception of dental auxiliaries is that they are very knowledgeable about dentistry, they do not have x-ray quotas to fill and they do not receive a bonus for exposing additional numbers of x-ray images. Therefore, a dental auxiliary is perceived as someone who can offer unbiased answers to their questions. Here are ten questions that a patient may ask their dental professional prior to being exposed to x-radiation. Each question is accompanied by a simple response that should educate and allay the fears of the patient.

1. How often should I get x rays taken?

Response: The frequency and type of dental x-ray images required will vary from one patient to another. This is because our mouths are all different. Someone who has never had a dental cavity in their entire life may only need a couple of bitewing x rays taken every few years to confirm that no problems have developed. While someone else who is very prone to tooth decay may need multiple x rays taken, for example every 6 months. Our office only takes the minimal number of x rays to ensure that you receive the best oral care.

2. How much radiation am I receiving from dental x rays?

Response: You may not realize it, but you are continually receiving a low dose of radiation from everything around you. Radiation comes from the sun, the ground you walk on, the buildings that surround you, etc. We call this

Fundamentals of Oral and Maxillofacial Radiology, First Edition. J. Sean Hubar.
© 2017 John Wiley & Sons, Inc. Published 2017 by John Wiley & Sons, Inc.
Companion website: www.wiley.com/go/hubar/radiology

natural background radiation. Our typical dental exam x rays amount to less than 1 day's worth of normal radiation and that is regardless of whether you are spending time indoors or outdoors in the sun all day. Do you ever travel in a plane? Flying in a plane at a higher altitude exposes you typically to more radiation than our dental x rays do. We also take all precautions to protect you from unnecessary radiation by using the latest technology.

3. Can I get cancer from dental x rays?

Response: Going back to the discovery of x rays in the late 1800s, there has not been one proven instance of a patient getting cancer from dental x rays. And today, with our improved technology, you receive far less radiation than dental patients did back in those early days.

4. Why do I need to wear a protective apron for dental x rays and why does the assistant leave the room before taking my x rays, if dental x rays are so safe?

Response: Our office prides itself on using whatever means we can to help reduce any unnecessary exposure both to you and to me. Our policy is: if it is simple to do, then we should do it. To protect you from x rays that may bounce off your teeth and jaws in different directions, I will place a protective apron on you, and to protect me from those same x rays, I will stand outside the room.

5. Your protective apron does not have a thyroid collar, why not?

Response: Depending on the type of x rays we require, the collar can actually get in the way of the x-ray beam and block the x rays making

it impossible to see your teeth and jaws on the image. If that happened, then we would have to expose you again, with the collar removed. So to avoid having to re-expose you, we leave it off when necessary. You may not realize it, but some of x rays that bounce off your teeth and bones exit your jaws through your neck. While you are wearing a thyroid collar, these x rays can actually bounce backward off the collar and expose your thyroid gland to additional x rays that would have just exited your body.

6. I am pregnant, should I get dental x rays taken?

Response: To be 100% safe, it is always best to avoid having any x-ray images taken at any stage of your pregnancy. Treating your dental problem is essential to the good health of your developing baby. If you have an untreated dental infection, more harm could result to the baby than by taking a few x rays and properly treating the problematic tooth. We will take the minimum number of x rays to treat that problem and we will take all precautions to reduce the radiation exposure to you and your baby. That means, to protect your baby, I will place a protective apron on you which will absorb over 99% of the few stray x rays that might bounce off your teeth and jaws. You and your baby will be fully protected.

7. When should my child first get dental x rays taken?

Response: It is vital to follow the development of the baby teeth and the developing adult teeth. Every child will react differently to having dental instruments placed in their mouths. Pediatric dentists recommend first seeing children at a few years of age. At that time, a minimal number of dental x rays may be attempted to properly examine a child's teeth.

8. Will I glow in the dark after all of the x rays that I received at the dental office?

Response: Never! Dental x rays do not make people glow regardless of the exposure dose. The "glowing" that you are referring to is related to radioactive materials found in nature. X rays are not radioactive.

9. What are 3-D x rays?

Response: In many dental offices today, there is a new type of sophisticated dental x-ray unit. It is called a *cone beam computed tomography* (CBCT) x-ray unit. It produces three-dimensional views of your jaws. It does not replace our standard x rays because the images do not show fine details well, like small cavities, and it requires more radiation exposure compared with standard x-ray images. However, it is invaluable for patients requiring dental implants. It is also used sometimes for cosmetic surgery, orthodontics, root canals and diagnosing pathology.

10. Why does the dentist require additional 3-D x rays before placing my dental implant?

Response: Standard dental x rays, like panoramic x rays, only show the outer surface of the bones and teeth in two dimensions and these x-ray images are somewhat distorted. It is not a technique error but rather it is a physical problem built into that type of x-ray equipment, which results in unavoidably distorted x rays of the teeth and bones. For successful implant placement, it is critical to have accurate images in all three dimensions showing the precise size and shape of the bone where the implant will be placed. CBCT provides us with this vital missing information. Cone beam images also accurately show the position of the nerve in the jaw so we can avoid damaging it when placing your dental implant.

Appendix 3
Helpful Tips for Difficult Patients

1. Hypersensitive gag reflex

A gag reflex is also termed a *pharyngeal reflex* or a *laryngeal spasm*. It is a reflexive contraction of the posterior region of the throat that includes the back of the tongue, the roof of the mouth and the tonsillar area. The gag reflex is typically triggered by tactile stimulation (i.e. physical contact). However, a patient's hypersensitive gag reflex may be triggered by the mere sight of an intraoral x-ray instrument. A hypersensitive gag reflex is of particular concern when performing intraoral imaging procedures. **(Note: Some people do not have any gag reflex, possibly due to a medical condition such as vagus or glossopharyngeal nerve damage.)**

The maxillary molar view is often the most problematic area for patients. If multiple regions of the mouth are to be imaged, the author recommends that the operator complete all of the other areas first and then return to image the maxillary molar region at the very end. If a patient is predisposed to gagging, starting in the maxillary molar region may stress the patient so much that it may be impossible to continue. A consequence of this might be the inability for the operator to image the anterior region of the mouth, an area that often does not trigger a gag reflex. If a full mouth series of images is required, then the operator should wait until nearing the end of the procedure to casually inform the patient that only a couple of maxillary molars remain. Knowing that only one or two images remain to be taken may allow the patient to persevere and briefly permit the operator to complete the series.

Most importantly, when faced with a patient having a hypersensitive gag reflex, the operator should perform the intraoral procedures as expeditiously as possible. That means pre-setting the exposure time, kilovoltage and milliamperage and pre-positioning the PID prior to inserting the receptor into the patient's mouth. In addition, only the operator should be in the room with the patient during the procedure. If other office personnel or family members are present to assist, they should be outside the operatory to avoid unnecessary delays clearing the room to permit immediate exposure once the receptor is inserted into the patient's mouth. Time is of the essence!

Utilizing the distal oblique technique might be advantageous in some cases (see Section K). Even though the distal oblique angulation will

Fundamentals of Oral and Maxillofacial Radiology, First Edition. J. Sean Hubar.
© 2017 John Wiley & Sons, Inc. Published 2017 by John Wiley & Sons, Inc.
Companion website: www.wiley.com/go/hubar/radiology

likely overlap images of the crowns, the periapical areas usually will be clearly visible. The crowns can then be visualized on bitewing images. In general, if bitewing images are prescribed in addition to periapical images, it is recommended that the bitewings always be imaged at the outset. Bitewing images are well tolerated by most patients and they offer additional information that is not evident in other views.

Distractions are useful ploys to counteract gagging. Instructing the patient to breathe deeply through their nose may calm and subdue the gag reflex. Additionally, instructing the patient to raise one arm and one leg prior to inserting the receptor has also been shown to help. The patient's need to concentrate on keeping an arm and a leg raised may offer enough distraction for the individual to forget about the instrumentation being placed intraorally.

More tangible remedies include swabbing both the hard and soft palate with a topical analgesic. This will temporarily anaesthetize the sensitive regions and generally allow placement of the intraoral instrument properly. Similarly, gargling with a mouth rinse or sprinkling salt on the patient's tongue immediately prior to instrument placement may also reduce a patient's gag reflex. If there is a trained individual in the dental office that can perform hypnosis on the patient and the patient is compliant, this may remedy a hypersensitive gag reflex to permit placement of the intraoral instrumentation.

If none of the remedies discussed above work, the operator should supplement any intraoral images acquired with extraoral imaging, such as a panoramic projection. Some newer panoramic units also claim to offer software to capture bitewing images. However the bitewing images attained with a panoramic unit will not be as diagnostic as conventional intraoral bitewing images simply due to using different geometric principles.

It is important to note that if a patient is intolerant at any time during the procedure, the operator should suggest terminating the procedure that day and attempting again on another day. The risk to the dental practice is that a traumatized patient may decide not to return to the office for future treatment.

2. Small mouth/shallow palate/constricted arch/torus

Solid-state digital receptors do not adapt well to situations where space is limited. The problem here is that current receptors are rigid and are relatively bulky in size. Patients with a narrow arch, shallow palate or mandible or the presence of a torus complicate proper placement of the receptor for performing the paralleling technique. Options for the operator are limited. Using a PSP plate is preferable in these scenarios. PSP plates are thinner and are flexible, much like dental x-ray film. Rarely will a dental practice have both solid-state and PSP receptors because of the high financial cost. PSP systems are currently unpopular with a majority of dentists because of the added time and steps required for scanning the individual PSP plates. If the operator uses a solid-state receptor, substituting a size 2 receptor with a smaller receptor size 1 or 0 should help. However, the operator should be aware that the smaller receptor is also shorter and that it may not be long enough to capture the length of the entire tooth on a single image. The operator should focus on the region of primary interest but take whatever images are necessary to perform a proper diagnosis.

A shallow palate necessitates using the bisecting angle technique. If the operator attempts performing the paralleling technique, it will likely result in a foreshortened image caused by excessive vertical angulation of the x-ray beam. The presence of a palatal torus in a deep palatal vault basically has the same effect as a shallow palate alone. Similarly, a shallow floor of the mouth (i.e. inadequate vertical height of the mandibular ridge) may prevent the operator from fully seating the receptor vertically to image the periapical region. A shallow palate and a shallow floor of the mouth are particularly common in children, simply because of incomplete growth and development. The fact is that it may be impossible to acquire diagnostic intraoral images on some patients and the practitioner must then rely strictly on extraoral images. As mentioned earlier, some panoramic units offer software to capture bitewing images but they will not be as diagnostic as conventional intraoral bitewing images.

3. Large frenulum

The lingual frenulum is a small fold of mucous membrane in the midline that extends from the floor of the mouth to the ventral surface of the tongue. A large lingual frenulum may restrict the ability of the patient to raise his or her tongue for the operator to properly position the intraoral receptor beneath it for the mandibular anterior periapical views. To counteract this problem, the operator may simply place the instrument on the dorsal surface of the tongue and have the patient fully close the jaws together. Generally, this will adequately capture the anterior periapical regions. Another option is for the operator to use the bisecting angle technique. In this case, the receptor should be positioned as far lingually as possible and the angulation of the x-ray beam can then be determined using the bisecting angle formula. Positioning the receptor in the posterior regions should not be affected by the lingual frenulum (synonym: frenum).

4. Trismus

Trismus is a spasm of the muscles of mastication that prevent the patient from opening his or her mouth appreciably. Insufficient opening of the mandible and maxilla may prevent insertion of the receptor instrumentation into the patient's mouth. Extraoral imaging may be the only method for imaging the teeth if the bulkiness of a solid-state receptor combined with the x-ray instrument is too large to insert. Without the convenience of extraoral imaging, the operator can remove the x-ray instrument and position the receptor itself horizontally onto the occlusal surfaces of the teeth and perform multiple occlusal technique views to acquire some intraoral images. If a PSP plate is available, the operator may substitute a hemostat for the standard instrument. A hemostat, being less bulky, would permit sliding the receptor horizontally between the teeth and, once inside the mouth, the receptor could be flipped upright and positioned apically. Depending on the final vertical orientation of the receptor, the bisecting angle or paralleling technique can then be used by the operator.

5. Cuspid superimposition

The position of the cuspid is normally situated along the anterior curvatures of both the maxilla and the mandible. The curve of either arch forces positioning the receptor obliquely behind the cuspid. The resultant horizontal angulation invariably projects the lingual cusp of the first premolar over the distal surface of the cuspid. Consequently, superimposition of the cuspid and first premolar contacts in the cuspid view is commonplace. However, the overlapped contacts between the cuspid and first premolar should ideally be open in the premolar periapical and bitewing images. One caveat here is that a solid-state receptor may be too bulky to be positioned far enough anteriorly to capture the distal of the cuspid. The operator can compromise by angling the receptor horizontally across the midline. This should position the receptor far enough anteriorly to capture and open the distal contact of the cuspid. However in this orientation, the horizontal angulation of the PID will likely produce some uneven magnification and overlapping of the two premolars.

Consequently, additional traditional premolar views would need to be imaged to complete the series.

6. Rubber dam

Dental procedures, such as endodontic or restorative treatments, typically involve the use of a rubber dam which will complicate intraoral receptor positioning. Regardless if the rubber dam frame is metal or plastic, it should be removed to facilitate placement of the receptor. Customized x-ray instruments are commercially available (e.g. Endo-Ray®) to accommodate the rubber dam, the rubber dam clamp and possible endodontic instruments. Other options may include using tongue depressors (see Figs Y12 and Y13) and hemostats. Hemostats should only be used with PSP plates and not solid-state receptors. All solid-state receptors are much thicker than PSP plates and may be damaged by tightly clamping the hemostat onto them. Generally, the bisecting angle technique must be used because the receptor cannot be positioned or maintained parallel to the tooth of interest. When necessary, patients may be requested to hold the x-ray instrument with their own hand because it may be physically impossible to occlude the teeth together to support the instrument.

7. Third molar imaging

Intraoral imaging of a third molar is often challenging for even an experienced operator. In addition, it is not uncommon for an unerupted third molar to be horizontally impacted. This will further compound the difficulty level in attempting to acquire an image of the entire tooth. Gagging often becomes an issue when placing receptors far enough posteriorly to image third molars, particularly maxillary third molars. Tips for treating gagging patients are discussed earlier in this appendix and may be used with some success in this situation. Alternatively, the distal oblique intraoral technique, also previously discussed, would be worth attempting. In this scenario, the receptor would only need to be positioned in the premolar region and then angled across the midline to capture the image. Ultimately it may be impossible to acquire an intraoral image of a third molar and an extraoral image such as a two-dimensional panoramic projection is the alternative. Besides the procedure being more comfortable for the patient, a panoramic projection will image all of the third molars simultaneously. A CBCT may alternatively be prescribed for obtaining the three-dimensional relationship of the third molars to their surrounding structures.

Appendix 4
Deficiencies of X-ray Imaging Terminology

Soap bubble, honeycomb and *multilocular* are terms frequently used interchangeably to describe similar radiologic features. Do these terms describe a single entity or are they characteristic of different osseous pathoses? The nomenclature used in dental radiology is confusing: the dental literature shows linguistic ambiguity and impreciseness. Descriptive terms selected to describe lesions of the jaws are often ill-defined or may possibly be undefined. Although *honeycomb* and *soap bubble* are frequently used interchangeably to describe the same ameloblastoma, the Concise English dictionary provides different definitions for the two descriptors. *Honeycomb* is defined as a "regular arrangement of numerous, small, uniform compartments," whereas *soap bubble* is described as "numerous, non-uniform compartments of varying size and arranged in an irregular pattern." Additional examples of ambiguous terminology presently in use include *lace-like, moth-eaten, worm-eaten, sun ray, sunburst, ground glass* and *cotton wool*.

To investigate this perceived problem in communication with current radiographic terminology, the author conducted a limited survey. The terms included in the study were *cotton wool, ground glass, honeycomb, multilocular* and *soap bubble*. Definitions for these terms were obtained from five oral and maxillofacial radiologists, an oral and maxillofacial surgeon, an attorney, two linguists and an English language professor.

Survey results

The following definitions were supplied by the ten respondents.

Cotton wool appearance (see Fig. X6)

Oral and maxillofacial radiologists:

1. Irregular, ill-defined radiopaque patches
2. Fluffy, rounded, opaque mass without distinct margins
3. Rounded radiopacities within an area of more radiolucent bone
4. Numerous foci of radiopacity intermingled with areas of radiolucency
5. Radiopaque globular or spherical structures with reduced numbers and thicknesses of trabeculae and haphazard or linear pattern of those that remain

Oral and maxillofacial surgeon: Like balls of cotton, fuzzy edges, centrally radiopaque

Attorney: Large, round, soft, puffy area, perhaps with soft wisps or tendrils; white or light in color relative to the background

Linguists:

1. Composed of a mass of fluffy white threads
2. Frothy white with no real shape except a general roundness; edges ill-defined

English professor: Spherical fibrous mass(es)

Ground glass appearance (see Fig. X3)

Oral and maxillofacial radiologists:

1. Fine, almost structureless granular texture; may be more or less radiopaque than normal
2. Granular radiographic appearance resembling an orange peel or pebbled texture; variable margin patterns
3. Homogeneous appearance of bone resulting from loss of contrast between trabeculae and marrow spaces
4. Appearance of glass with light-diffusing surface produced by etching or *abrasion* ☢ (i.e. hazy, filmy appearance); many trabeculae of bone of approximately equal size are radiographically apparent
5. Resembling glass which has been pulverized into fine granules

Oral and maxillofacial surgeon: Amorphous radiopaque appearance

Attorney: Evenly sized small compact grains

Linguists:

1. Composed of tiny, hard, shiny particles
2. Fairly flat and composed of small hard bits resembling granulated sugar

English professor: Crystalline-appearance of chunks with hard edges

Honeycomb appearance (see Fig. X5)

Oral and maxillofacial radiologists:

1. Multilocular lesion with compartments smaller than those of "soap bubble" appearance
2. Contiguous polygonal radiolucent regions, which may vary in border definition
3. Numerous small compartments with septal arrangement resembling a honeycomb
4. Similar to "multilocular" but with more linear septae
5. Not used and no opinion

Oral and maxillofacial surgeon: Not used

Attorney: Well-defined, roughly similar, round or squarish geometric areas branching out over relatively wide areas; separate shapes appear empty

Linguists:

1. Composed of regularly joined polygons
2. Framework of adjoining octagonally-shaped hollow cells

English professor: Hexagonal structures

Multilocular appearance (see Fig. X1)

Oral and maxillofacial radiologists:

1. Radiolucency produced by many coalescing and overlapping compartments in bone; often representative of a neoplastic or cystic process
2. Radiolucency with more than one locule, having many compartments
3. Usually pathologic well-corticated radiolucencies; internal septae, total or partially separate compartments (in two-dimensions) within the boundaries of the lesion
4. Radiolucent lesion with two or more round or ovoid compartments which appear to be

partially separated from one another by incomplete septae

5. Having many compartments

Oral and maxillofacial surgeon: Multicystic or soap bubble appearance

Attorney: Many circles in a well-defined area

Linguists:

1. Unknown
2. Unknown

English professor: Spheres or ovals within a larger body

Soap bubble appearance (see Fig. X1)

Oral and maxillofacial radiologists:

1. Multilocular lesion consisting of several circular compartments which vary in size and usually appear to be somewhat overlapped
2. Multilocular radiolucency with many locules varying in size from large to very small
3. Radiolucent compartments of variable size, faint septae and poorly defined borders
4. Similar to "multilocular" but with more rounded septae
5. Similar to "multilocular" but with many loculations; reminiscent of soap bubbles; bony septae between locules are very fine whereas in "multilocular" lesions the septae can be coarse

Oral and maxillofacial surgeon: Multilocular with compartments of varying size

Attorney: Many small spheres clustered together; light density, puffy and soft, and empty or clear in appearance

Linguists:

1. Composed of mass of iridescent spheres of numerous sizes
2. Large shiny balls, each ball or sphere impinging on and partially adhering to other balls or spheres

English professor: Cluster of spherical masses with flat adjoining surfaces (i.e. with mutual walls)

Examination of the definitions just listed shows the discrepancies in the respondents' perceptions. Hence it is apparent that terms currently used by dental professionals to describe x-ray images are ambiguous. Interpretation is based on individuals' own conceptions and past education. Such impreciseness could lead to a gap in communication of significance to patient treatment and outcome.

Gill *et al.* (1973) evaluated observer variations in history taking and physical examination. He found disagreement was significantly reduced when a common set of definitions was developed and used by the participating physicians. It is suggested that a standardized set of definitions of radiographic features, if formulated, could reduce the margin of error currently resulting from subjective interpretation and definitional variability among dental diagnosticians.

Appendix 5
Tools for Differential Diagnosis

There are seven criteria useful for describing osseous lesions to formulate a differential diagnosis:

1. Number
2. Location
3. Density
4. Shape
5. Size
6. Borders
7. Changes to surrounding anatomic structures such as root resorption and tooth displacement

Note: Each criterion listed above has limited value on its own, but a combination of all seven can significantly improve the differential diagnosis. Ultimately a biopsy of the lesion may still be required to confirm the diagnosis.

1. Number

How many anomalies are present? Excluding tooth-specific pathology (e.g. caries) and generalized pathology (e.g. metabolic disease) that may encompass one or both dental arches entirely, the vast majority of osseous lesions appear single in number. Consequently, when a couple or more lesions are observed, it can assist the clinician in narrowing down the differential diagnosis. For example, bilateral radiolucencies in the rami of young individuals are very characteristic for cherubism.

2. Location

Where is the anomaly located? Is it in a tooth-bearing region or a non-tooth-bearing region? This information can help to differentiate odontogenic versus non-odontogenic pathology from the diagnosis. Many types of osseous pathology characteristically occur in one region of the mandible or maxilla. However, with the paucity of cases reported in the dental literature for some types of pathology, one must not eliminate an entity because it is located in a non-characteristic region of the facial complex. Location often helps to rank diagnoses higher or lower in the differential depending on whether it is found within or outside of its typical region.

Fundamentals of Oral and Maxillofacial Radiology, First Edition. J. Sean Hubar.
© 2017 John Wiley & Sons, Inc. Published 2017 by John Wiley & Sons, Inc.
Companion website: www.wiley.com/go/hubar/radiology

3. Density

Is the anomaly radiolucent, radiopaque or mixed (i.e. combination of radiolucent and radiopaque)? Density is invaluable for discerning the composition of the anomaly. Radiolucent areas typically indicate a destructive process within the area in question. Excluding an air space, radiolucent areas will be composed of soft tissue, fluids or a combination of the two. A radiopaque area typically indicates a calcifying (i.e. ossifying) process. A mixed radiolucent and radiopaque region may be either a destructive process or a calcifying process. For example, osteomyelitis is an infection leading to destruction of bone. While an ossifying fibroma is a calcifying process that may show both radiopaque and radiolucent regions during its intermediate stage of development. Interestingly, one must be cognizant about soft tissue and fluids located within more radiolucent areas of the orofacial complex (e.g. sinus). Contrary to what one would expect, in this situation soft tissue and fluids will not appear radiolucent but rather will have a somewhat radiopaque appearance. The reason is that soft tissue and fluids will attenuate additional radiation, giving it a radiopaque appearance relative to a less dense surrounding region. If the same soft tissue or fluid was located within a more opaque region like the ramus, it would typically appear radiolucent. Density is the most important finding for deriving a differential diagnosis.

4. Shape

Is the area in question, for example, round, elliptical, square or amorphous? Quite often, shape is used to characteristically describe the typical appearance of a particular disease process. *Soap bubble* ♠ appearance is often associated with an ameloblastoma; *honeycomb* ♠ appearance is often associated with a myxoma; *sunburst* ♠ appearance is associated with an

osteosarcoma, etc. The problem is that these radiologic terms are rarely defined in publications, leaving the interpretation up to the observer. More importantly, these appearances often only appear in the late stages of disease development. As a result, observing an earlier stage of disease development, the lesion may appear very different and the clinician may incorrectly discard that disease entity from the differential diagnosis because it did not have the classic radiologic appearance.

Shape indirectly can assist the clinician in assessing the consistency of the lesion. A round radiolucency would be more indicative of a fluid core. The dynamics of a round-shaped radiolucency is similar to a balloon. As the balloon inflates and as the radiolucency enlarges, they expand evenly in all directions. Of course shape exceptions will occur when an enlarging radiolucent area encounters an obstacle, e.g. a root of a tooth. The obstacle can act as a barrier and force the expanding lesion to detour around it, thus altering the symmetric shape. Conversely, an irregular-shaped radiolucency not modified by other structures might be more indicative of a soft tissue composition. Similar to flowers budding on a stem of a plant, a soft tissue lesion may bud out in different directions.

5. Size

How large is the area of concern? Size can be a general indicator of the period of time the lesion has been developing. One would generally expect that a larger lesion would have required a longer period of time to grow. A large lesion could also imply that it is benign in nature, particularly if it is painless. If the lesion was painful, it is more likely that the patient would have sought treatment earlier when the lesion was smaller in size. A great deal of weight should not be applied to this interpretation (i.e. benign versus malignant), but combined with all the other findings, it may help to modify the differential diagnosis.

For the differential diagnosis, size does not have to be 100% accurate. However, descriptive terms such as *large*, *big* and *small* are all too subjective and as a result should not be used by clinicians. Each person may interpret these terms very differently. If you are consulting with another clinician over the telephone about a case, it is best to describe the size of the area using either an approximate numeric measurement or simply comparing its size to a commonly known object (e.g. size of a dime) that others will be familiar with. This will better assist the other clinician to mentally envision the lesion.

6. Borders

Is the area well-demarcated, does it have a corticated border, is it difficult to differentiate abnormal from normal tissue? Well-defined borders are typically indicative of a slower growing, non-malignant lesion versus an ill-defined lesion. An ill-defined lesion would be more indicative of an aggressive, possibly malignant lesion. Well-corticated borders are indicative of the body's attempt at curtailing the lesion's growth; in essence the body's defense is attempting to wall it off. Aggressive, rapidly growing lesions will not be easily contained, will spread around obstacles (e.g. teeth) and will often appear with ill-defined borders. Be certain not to confuse ill-defined borders with poor diagnostic quality x-ray images.

7. Changes to surrounding anatomic structures

Radiographic changes such as expansion of the cortical plate, root resorption and tooth displacement are useful for determining the behavior of the lesion. Expansion of the cortical plate versus destruction of it is indicative of a slower-growing, less aggressive lesion. Root resorption is indicative of a slower-growing or long-standing lesion because of the time it would take to cause destruction of a solid tooth structure. Pathologic tooth displacement, like orthodontic tooth movement, is not a quick process. It would indicate a slower-growing lesion. A rapidly growing lesion would quickly spread around the tooth. Consequently, changes to normal anatomic structures are worth noting to help ascertain the behavior of the lesion in question.

In conclusion, combining all of the information from the seven criteria discussed above will give the clinician a significant amount of information to help construct a concise differential diagnosis. This is especially critical in a private practice scenario when the clinician has a patient who presents with some unknown oral pathology. The practice may not have advanced imaging modalities like CBCT or have a pathologist's biopsy report at the initial visit. Yet the patient expects some information about the seriousness of the situation before departing the dental office. Fortunately, the clinician can dissect significant amounts of information from conventional x-ray images and combine that with information derived from the medical history and dental exam to give the patient an intelligent answer as to the behavior of the lesion and how to proceed. It may or may not be enough information to accurately diagnose the lesion but at least the behavior of the pathosis should be evident.

Appendix 6
Table of Radiation Units

Traditional units	SI units	Conversion
Roentgen (R)	Coulombs per kilogram (C/kg)	2.58×10^{-4} C/kg = 1 R
Radiation absorbed dose (rad)	Gray (Gy)	1 Gy = 100 rad
Roentgen equivalent man (rem)	Sievert (Sv)	1 Sv = 100 rem

Fundamentals of Oral and Maxillofacial Radiology, First Edition. J. Sean Hubar.
© 2017 John Wiley & Sons, Inc. Published 2017 by John Wiley & Sons, Inc.
Companion website: www.wiley.com/go/hubar/radiology

Appendix 7
Table of Anatomic Landmarks

Tooth

- Dentin
- Cementum
- Enamel
- Pulp

Tooth-related structures

- Alveolar bone (cancellous and cortical bone)
- Alveolar crest
- Lamina dura
- Periodontal ligament space

Landmarks associated with the maxilla

Radiopaque

- Anterior nasal spine
- Hamular process
- Nasal concha
- Nasolabial fold
- Nose (soft tissue)
- Pterygoid plates
- Torus (aka palatine torus, torus palatinus; pl. tori)
- Zygoma and zygomatic process

Radiolucent

- Incisive foramen
- Lateral fossa
- Lip line
- Maxillary sinus
- Mid-palatine suture (aka intermaxillary suture)
- Nasal fossa
- Nasolacrimal canal

Landmarks associated with the mandible

Radiopaque

- Coronoid process
- Genial tubercles

Fundamentals of Oral and Maxillofacial Radiology, First Edition. J. Sean Hubar.
© 2017 John Wiley & Sons, Inc. Published 2017 by John Wiley & Sons, Inc.
Companion website: www.wiley.com/go/hubar/radiology

- Inferior border of the mandible
- Lip line (soft tissue)
- Mental ridge (aka mental process)
- Oblique ridge, external
- Oblique ridge, internal
- Torus (aka mandibular torus, torus mandibularis; pl. tori)

Radiolucent

- Lingual foramen
- Mandibular canal
- Mental foramen
- Mental fossa
- Nutrient canals
- Submandibular gland fossa

Appendix 8
Table of Dental Anomalies

Number

- Anodontia
- Oligodontia
- Supernumerary tooth

Size

- Macrodontia
- Microdontia

Shape

- Concrescence
- Dens evaginatus
- Dens invaginatus
- Denticle
- Dentinal bridge
- Dilaceration
- Enamel pearl
- Fusion
- Gemination
- Hutchinson's incisor
- Hypercementosis
- Mulberry molar
- Taurodont tooth
- Turner's tooth

Developmental defects

- Dysplasia, dentin
- Hypoplasia, enamel
- Imperfecta, amelogenesis
- Imperfecta, dentinogenesis
- Imperfecta, osteogenesis
- Odontodysplasia, regional
- Pulpal obliteration

Environmental effects

- Abrasion
- Ankylosis
- Attrition
- Calculus
- Caries, dental
- Caries, radiation
- Erosion
- Foreign body
- Fracture
- Impaction
- Resorption, external
- Resorption, internal
- Restorations
- Rotation
- Transposition

Fundamentals of Oral and Maxillofacial Radiology, First Edition. J. Sean Hubar.
© 2017 John Wiley & Sons, Inc. Published 2017 by John Wiley & Sons, Inc.
Companion website: www.wiley.com/go/hubar/radiology

Appendix 9
Table of Osseous Pathology

Radiolucent anomalies in the maxilla and mandible

- Abscess, periapical
- Ameloblastoma
- Bone marrow defect
- Calcifying epithelial odontogenic tumor (early stage)
- Cherubism
- Cysts:
  - aneurysmal bone
  - botryoid
  - calcifying odontogenic
  - dentigerous
  - incisive canal
  - lateral periodontal
  - median palatine
  - nasopalatine
  - odontogenic keratocyst (see *keratinizing odontogenic tumor*)
  - periapical (radicular)
  - residual
  - Stafne bone
  - traumatic bone
- Fibrosarcoma
- Fibrous dysplasia (early stage)
- Florid osseous dysplasia (early stage)
- Giant cell granuloma
- Giant cell tumor
- Granuloma, periapical
- Hemangioma
- Hyperparathyroidism
- Keratinizing odontogenic tumor
- Metastatic tumor
- Multiple myeloma
- Myxoma
- Osseous dysplasia (early stage)
- Ossifying fibroma (early stage)
- Osteoporosis
- Salivary gland tumors, benign and malignant
- Scar, periapical

Radiopaque anomalies in the maxilla and mandible

- Antrolith (located within a sinus)
- Calcifying epithelial odontogenic tumor (late stage)
- Cementoblastoma
- Condensing osteitis
- Enostosis
- Exostosis
- Fibrous dysplasia (late stage)
- Florid osseous dysplasia (late stage)

Fundamentals of Oral and Maxillofacial Radiology, First Edition. J. Sean Hubar.
© 2017 John Wiley & Sons, Inc. Published 2017 by John Wiley & Sons, Inc.
Companion website: www.wiley.com/go/hubar/radiology

- Foreign body
- Odontoma: complex, compound
- Osseous dysplasia (late stage)
- Ossifying fibroma (late stage)
- Osteopetrosis
- Phleboliths, intraoral
- Torus: palatine, mandibular

Mixed (radiolucent–radiopaque) anomalies in the maxilla and mandible

- Calcifying epithelial odontogenic cyst
- Calcifying epithelial odontogenic tumor (intermediate stage)

- Condensing osteitis
- Fibrosarcoma (intermediate stage)
- Fibrous dysplasia (intermediate stage)
- Osseous dysplasia (intermediate stage)
- Ossifying fibroma (intermediate stage)
- Osteomyelitis
- Osteosarcoma
- Paget's disease
- Periapical osseous dysplasia (intermediate stage)

Appendix 10
Common Abbreviations and Acronyms

☢ is the universal symbol for radiation that is posted in public areas where there is ionizing radiation in the immediate vicinity.

A	amp/amperage
ADA	American Dental Association
AIDS	acquired immunodeficiency syndrome
ALADA	as low as diagnostically acceptable
ALARA	as low as reasonably achievable
BID	beam indicating device
BOC	botryoid odontogenic cyst
BW	bitewing
CBCT	cone beam computed tomography
CCD	charge coupled device
CDC	Centers for Disease Control and Prevention
CEOT	calcifying epithelial odontogenic tumor
cm	centimeter
CMOS	complementary metal oxide semiconductor
CMX	complete mouth series of x rays
COC	calcifying odontogenic cyst
CT	computed tomography
DHCP	dental healthcare practitioner
DICOM	digital imaging and communications in medicine
EM	electromagnetic
EPA	Environmental Protection Agency
FDA	Food and Drug Administration
FMS or FMX	full mouth series of x rays
FOV	field of view
Gy	gray
HBV	hepatitis B virus
HIPAA	Health Information Portability and Accountability Act
HIV	human immunodeficiency virus
HVL	half value layer
Hz	hertz
ICRP	International Commission on Radiological Protection
kerma	kinetic energy released per unit mass

Fundamentals of Oral and Maxillofacial Radiology, First Edition. J. Sean Hubar.
© 2017 John Wiley & Sons, Inc. Published 2017 by John Wiley & Sons, Inc.
Companion website: www.wiley.com/go/hubar/radiology

kV	kilovolt/kilovoltage	**PDL**	periodontal ligament
kVp	kilovolt peak	**PID**	position indicating device
LPC	lateral periodontal cyst	**PPE**	personal protection equipment
mA	milliamp/milliamperage	**PSP**	photostimulable phosphor
mAs	milliampere seconds	**QA**	quality assurance
MPD	maximum permissible dose	**R**	roentgen
MPR	multiplanar reconstruction	**rad**	radiation absorbed dose
MRI	magnetic resonance imaging	**rem**	radiation or roentgen equivalent man
mSv	millisievert		
NCRP	National Council on Radiation Protection and Measurements	**RHI**	receptor holding instrument
		SI	*Système Internationale* or international system of units
nm	nanometer		
OSHA	Occupational Safety and Health Administration	**SLOB**	same–lingual, opposite–buccal
		TMD	temporomandibular joint dysfunction
PA	periapical image or the anteroposterior direction of an x-ray beam	**Sv**	sievert
		V	volt/voltage

Appendix 11
Glossary of Terms

Abrasion: the pathologic wearing of a tooth structure by mechanical means.

Absent crown: a tooth lacking its entire crown; the presence of roots only (e.g. radiation caries can preclude total crown destruction).

Absorption, x-ray: the attenuation of x-ray photon energy as it passes through a material.

ALADA: an acronym meaning "**as** **l**ow **as** **d**iagnostically **a**cceptable." The intent of this updated ALARA principle is for the operator to use a minimal dose of radiation exposure and still acquire a diagnostic image.

ALARA: an acronym meaning "**as** **l**ow **as** **r**easonably **a**chievable." The intent of this principle is for the operator to employ all reasonable measures to minimize a patient's exposure to radiation (e.g. use of a protective apron).

Alpha radiation: a form of particulate radiation emitted from heavy metals. It contains two protons and two neutrons identical to a helium nucleus. It is not able to penetrate skin.

Alveolar bone: the bone that comprises both the maxilla and the mandible. It surrounds the roots of teeth. The alveolar process is the specific region of bone that surrounds the roots of teeth and the sockets of missing teeth.

Amalgam: an alloy of metals which include mercury, silver, tin and copper. It has largely been replaced with non-metallic composite materials today. Amalgam restorations appear very radiopaque on dental images.

Ampere: represents the amount of current flowing in a circuit. One milliampere (mA) is one-thousandth of an amp. It primarily controls the quantity of radiation produced. Higher amperage results in a higher output of radiation from the x-ray tubehead.

Analog: x-ray film is considered to be an analog format. When the film, which is a polyester-base coated with a photosensitive emulsion, is exposed to radiation, it creates an analog image of an area of the dentition. Digital has largely replaced film as an image recording format.

Fundamentals of Oral and Maxillofacial Radiology, First Edition. J. Sean Hubar.
© 2017 John Wiley & Sons, Inc. Published 2017 by John Wiley & Sons, Inc.
Companion website: www.wiley.com/go/hubar/radiology

Angled root: a marked angulation of a root of a tooth in relation to its crown. Synonym: dilaceration.

Angström (Å): a unit of measure equaling one ten-billionth of a meter (10^{-10} m).

Angulation, horizontal: the side to side aiming direction of the PID. Proper horizontal angle is critical for exposing good bitewing images. Aiming the x-ray beam between adjacent tooth contacts is considered proper horizontal angulation. This should produce dental images with little or no overlap of interproximal contacts, which is important for diagnosing caries.

Angulation, vertical: the up and down aiming direction of the PID. Excessive vertical angulation (i.e. overangulation) will result in a foreshortened image, while insufficient vertical angulation (i.e. underangulation) will produce elongation of the image.

Anode: consists of a copper tube and a small tungsten focal spot. It is the positively-charged target end of the x-ray tube. High-speed electrons from the cathode strike the anode and produce quantities of x-ray photons.

Anodontia: the complete absence of all teeth is called *total anodontia*, while *partial anodontia* is the absence of some teeth.

Anterior loop of the mandibular canal: the mandibular canal forms the anterior loop by extending anteriorly beyond the mental foramen and then turning posteriorly to reach the mental foramen.

Anterior nasal spine: a small bony projection of the maxilla at the anterior aspect of the mid-palatine suture (i.e. anteroinferior aspect of the nasal cavity). It is often used as an orthodontic landmark on cephalographic images.

Antiseptic: an antimicrobial substance for reducing the potential for infection.

Aplasia: the congenital absence or abnormal development of a structure.

Atomic number: the number of protons within the nucleus of an atom.

Attenuation: the reduction in the intensity of the x-ray beam.

Attrition: the pathologic wearing down of a tooth structure by tooth to tooth contact.

Autoclaving: the use of high-pressure saturated steam to sterilize equipment.

Axial plane: an imaginary line that divides the patient's head into superior and inferior parts. It is perpendicular to the coronal and sagittal planes. Clinicians routinely view CBCT images in this perspective.

Background radiation: the ubiquitous environmental radiation that all people are exposed to on a daily basis. It includes both natural and artificial sources (e.g. cosmic rays, radon gas, nuclear fallout, occupational exposure). Background radiation levels will vary geographically depending on altitude and soil composition.

Barrier, protective: a physical mechanism to protect a patient or operator from contact with potentially infective substances such as blood and saliva. A *physical shield* is for the operator to stand behind for protection from stray x rays. A *barrier envelope* is a disposable plastic cover that slips over a dental receptor.

Beta radiation: beta particles are electron particles emitted from a nucleus; particulate radiation is unlike electromagnetic radiation, which has no mass.

BID: the acronym for **b**eam **i**ndicating **d**evice. (See PID.)

Bifid canal: the presence of a second mandibular canal running parallel to the primary mandibular canal. It houses smaller accessory branches of the inferior alveolar nerve. A bifid canal is more commonly seen in panoramic and CBCT images.

Bisect: divide into two equal size sections.

Bisecting angle technique: an intraoral imaging technique in which the operator bisects the angle formed by the long dimension of the tooth and the position of the receptor. The central x-ray beam is then aimed perpendicular to that imaginary line referred to as a bisector.

Bisphosphonates: a category of drugs prescribed for slowing down or preventing bone loss. They are commonly used to treat osteoporosis and cancers that affect bone mass (e.g. lung, breast and prostate tumors). Performing invasive dental procedures such as an extraction, an implant placement or endodontic surgery on a patient receiving long-term intravenously administered bisphosphonates has been linked to osteoradionecrosis. Diabetes has also been associated with *bisphosphonate osteonecrosis* ☢.

Bitewing image: an intraoral image that shows both the mandibular and maxillary crowns in one image. It is useful for diagnosing interproximal dental caries and alveolar bone height. Orientation of the long dimension of the image receptor sideways is referred to as a *horizontal bitewing;* orientation of the long dimension of the receptor upright is referred to as a *vertical bitewing*. Vertical bitewings are often preferred by periodontists to image more of the alveolar bone surrounding the teeth.

Bitewing tab: a simple intraoral receptor holding device usually made of paper or plastic for a patient to bite upon. It functions to secure the receptor in position for bitewing images. This allows the operator more flexibility in determining the correct horizontal angulation for avoiding overlapped interproximal contacts. It is particularly beneficial when there is tooth rotation or crowding present.

Botryoid: appearing like a cluster of grapes (e.g. botryoid odontogenic cyst).

Bregma: commonly referred to as the *soft spot* on the top of a newborn baby's head. It is the landmark on the skull where the sagittal and coronal sutures join and the parietal and frontal bones come together.

Bremsstrahlung radiation: a German term meaning *braking rays*. Bremsstrahlung radiation occurs when electrons collide with the anode in an x-ray tube. Virtually all x rays produced within the range of kilovoltage used in dental x-ray units are bremsstrahlung x rays. More powerful medical x-ray generators can additionally produce *characteristic radiation*.

Brightness: a measure of intensity after the image has been acquired.

Burnout: see Cervical burnout.

Bus, computer: a pathway that a computer uses to transfer data.

Café au lait spots: flat pigmented spots on the skin, the color of coffee with milk, commonly associated with fibrous dysplasia and neurofibromatosis.

Caries: see Dental caries.

Cathode: the negatively-charged end containing a tungsten filament within a dental x-ray tube. Heating the filament releases a cloud of electrons that can be accelerated across the tube to the anode to generate x rays.

CBCT: see cone beam computed tomography.

CCD (charge coupled device): a solid-state digital image receptor introduced into dentistry in 1987; basically it consists of a silicon wafer coated with a scintillation layer which increases the efficiency of x-ray absorption.

Central ray: for directional purposes, this refers to the x-ray stream that is located at the center of the beam as it exits from the PID.

Cephalograph: a lateral x-ray image of the skull showing both the bony and soft tissue structures. A head-positioning device referred to as a *cephalostat* is used for standardization and reproducibility. A cephalograph is typically used in orthodontic treatment to assess facial growth.

Cephalostat: a head-holding attachment on extraoral x-ray units for acquiring cephalograph images.

Cervical burnout: an illusionary radiolucency along the neck (i.e. cervical region) of the tooth caused by differential x-ray absorption. The dentin in the crown of the tooth is encapsulated with enamel; the dentin and cementum in the root of the tooth is surrounded by alveolar bone; the cervical region between the two is limited to only dentin and cementum. Consequently, more x rays penetrate through the cervical area, giving it a more radiolucent appearance compared to the encapsulated crown or the root embedded within bone. Cervical burnout can form a radiolucent band extending mesio-distally across the entire tooth or it may be localized to smaller areas in the mesial and/or distal surfaces along the neck of the tooth. It should not be misdiagnosed as dental caries.

Characteristic radiation: radiation that is produced when an electron is ejected from its orbit and another electron takes its place by dropping down from a higher shell. Dental x-ray units, unlike medical x-ray units, typically will not generate a kilovoltage great enough to produce characteristic radiation.

CMOS (complementary metal oxide semiconductor): a solid-state direct digital image receptor incorporating silicon based semiconductors. CMOS differs from CCD technology in how the charges produced by the absorbed x-ray photons are read. It is widely used in the manufacture of computer processing chips.

Collimation/collimator: All dental x-ray tubeheads contain a lead collimator to regulate the size and shape of an x-ray beam. A collimator is the device that will produce either a round or rectangular-shaped x-ray beam. The National Council on Radiation Protection and Measurements recommends using rectangular collimation. An advantage of rectangular collimation is an additional reduction in patient exposure compared to using round collimation. It is possible to convert a round beam into a rectangular collimated beam. A rectangular collimator can be attached to either the open end of a round PID or directly onto a receptor instrument itself. Regardless of the beam shape, beam size is government regulated. The maximum allowable size of an x-ray beam at the patient's face is 7 cm.

Complete dentition: the presence of a full complement of teeth.

Complete mouth series (CMX): see Full mouth series.

Compton scatter: this occurs when an incoming x-ray photon knocks out an orbiting electron from an outer shell of an atom. The net result is a positively charged atom and a free electron. The incoming x-ray photon gives up some of its energy and is redirected (i.e. scattered). The ejection of the electron from its orbit is referred to as *ionization* and the radiation itself is classified as *ionizing radiation*.

Concha: a horizontal outgrowth on the lateral wall of the nasal fossa. The nasal fossa has inferior, medial and superior conchae bilaterally. Synonym: turbinate.

Cone beam computed tomography (CBCT): CBCT technology was first introduced in 1996. Similar to a panoramic x-ray unit, a CBCT scanner rotates around the patient's head. However, unlike a panoramic unit, a CBCT unit acquires upwards of 600 individual images using a cone-shaped beam of x radiation. The acquired data is then reconstructed by a computer algorithm into axial, sagittal and coronal planar images.

Cone-cut: an intraoral technique error produced when an x-ray beam and a receptor are not properly matched with each other. The cone-cut is the blank area on the image that corresponds to the receptor area that was unexposed.

Conical: tapered; narrowing to a point.

Constricted: narrowed.

Contact, interproximal: refers to the contacting surfaces of two adjacent teeth. Bitewing images are intended to open adjacent tooth surfaces to primarily reveal the presence of caries. When adjacent tooth surfaces are superimposed upon one another, they are referred to as *overlapped contacts*. Incorrect horizontal angulation of the PID generally is the cause of overlapped contacts.

Contralateral side: affecting or occurring on the opposite side.

Contrast: refers to the degree of gray scale (i.e. number of shades of gray) differentiation that exists on an x-ray image. High-contrast images display fewer shades of gray than those of lower contrast. High-contrast images are better for visualizing dental caries, while low-contrast images are better for diagnosing periodontal conditions, such as crestal bone height. High contrast may be referred to as a *short-scale* contrast and low contrast is referred to as a *long-scale* contrast.

Coronal plane: a vertical plane that divides the body into anterior and posterior sections. Synonym: frontal plane.

Cortical plate, mandibular: the outer layer of compact bone that overlies the spongiosa bone of the alveolar process. It generally appears as a thin radiopaque line on x-ray images. Thinning of the cortical plates occurs naturally with age, but extreme thinning may also be the result of a metabolic disorder such as osteoporosis.

Cotton wool appearance: the alteration in trabeculae resulting in irregular patches of bone with increased density and diffuse borders resembling mycelium. These patchy areas, within which it is impossible to see any normal anatomic structures, may be a few millimeters to several centimeters in diameter. (See Fig. X6.)

Coulomb per kilogram (C/kg): the SI unit for ionizing radiation exposure. It is a measure of the amount of radiation required to create 1 C of charge in 1 kg of matter; 1 C/kg = 3875.96899224806 roentgen.

Crookes–Hittorf tube: a partially evacuated electrical discharge glass tube containing a cathode and an anode that can produce x-radiation when high voltage is applied to it. It was used by Professor Wilhelm Röntgen in 1895 when he discovered x rays. Modern vacuum x-ray tubes contain a heated filament (i.e. cathode) that release electrons.

Curve of Spee: the natural curvature of the mandibular occlusal plane beginning at the tip of the cuspid and continuing along the cusps of the posterior teeth.

Dead space, receptor: the inactive peripheral portion of a solid-state intraoral receptor that cannot capture an image.

Dens evaginatus: an enamel-covered tubercle that projects from the occlusal surface of an otherwise normal tooth. There is no age or sex predilection. The tubercle appears as a small, round radiopacity having the same density as enamel. Clinically, the evagination varies from one to several millimeters in size. The patient often presents with malocclusion and occlusal trauma.

Dens invaginatus: a developmental anomaly believed to arise from an invagination in the surface of the crown of a permanent tooth before calcification has occurred. The maxillary lateral incisors are most frequently affected. It often appears·as a pear-shaped radiolucent invagination lined with a thin layer of enamel and dentin that projects into the pulp. Synonym: dens in dente.

Density, image: the degree of darkness of an image. The brightness control in digital software programs controls image density.

Dental caries: demineralization of a calcified tooth structure results in the formation of a radiolucent area on an x-ray image. Synonyms: cavity or tooth decay.

Denticle: a round- or oval-shaped calcified body within a pulp chamber of either a permanent or deciduous tooth.

Dermatitis: a general term describing inflammation of the skin. It typically is a response to radiotherapy.

Deterministic effects: a minimum threshold dose of radiation exposure has to be surpassed for an effect to be observed. Severity of the effect is dose dependent. The higher the radiation dose received, the greater is the effect. Examples include erythema, epilation (i.e. hair loss), cataracts, etc. Synonym: non-stochastic effects. (See Stochastic effects.)

Diabetes mellitus, radiologic: uncontrolled diabetic patients often exhibit periodontal disease. In addition, diabetes may be a risk factor for developing bisphosphonate osteonecrosis.

DICOM (Digital Imaging and Communications in Medicine): a standard for handling, storing and transmitting information in digital images universally. DICOM includes a file format and a network communications protocol. These files can be exchanged between two entities that are capable of receiving image and patient data in a DICOM format.

Dilaceration: an angular distortion in the root or crown of a formed tooth. As a result, the tooth appears bent or twisted.

Direct digital receptor: an acquired image sent directly to a computer either via a wired receptor or via Wi-Fi transmission. Typically the receptor uses either CMOS or CCD technologies.

Disinfection: to destroy or inhibit the growth of pathogenic microorganisms by physical or chemical means.

Distortion, image: an exaggeration in the size and/or shape of an object on an x-ray image. A proper paralleling technique minimizes both size and shape distortion of intraoral images.

Dosimetry badge: a badge worn for recording cumulative x-radiation dose to personnel in the workplace. Government regulates occupational radiation exposure limits. Multiple companies offer monitoring services for dental office personnel for nominal fees. Synonym: dosimeter.

Duty cycle: the recommended time delay between x-ray exposures. Proper cooling of the x-ray tube is necessary to prolong the life expectancy of the x-ray tube. The life of the x-ray tube will be shortened if it is unable to cool down properly between exposures. Manufacturers of dental x-ray units provide duty cycle information for comparison shopping.

Ectodermal dysplasia: a group of genetic disorders of ectodermal structures. There may be abnormal development of the hair, teeth, nails and sweat glands.

Ectopic location: any tooth or object that is in an abnormal position.

Edentulous: the absence of one or more teeth.

Effective dose: the dose of ionizing radiation used to determine the probability of inducing genetic effects and cancer. It also allows the comparison of the effects of different types of radiation upon different types of tissues. The unit of effective dose is the sievert. *Effective dose equivalent* was shortened to "effective dose" in 1991.

Eggshell appearance: a thin, radiopaque, lamina-dura like layer of bone circumscribing either an oval-shaped radiolucent area or a radiolucent border around a radiopaque lesion.

Electromagnetic radiation: a form of energy that travels in wave form and has no mass. Examples include x rays, visible light, radio waves and microwaves.

Electron: a subatomic particle with a negative charge.

Electron cloud: the area around the heated cathode filament in an x-ray tube where free electrons congregate. Powering on an x-ray unit sends a low voltage current to the cathode of the x-ray tube. The filament heats up and emits electrons which remain at the cathode until the operator presses the exposure button. Depressing the exposure button sends a high voltage across the x-ray tube. This causes an acceleration of the electrons across to the anode and the generation of x-ray photons.

Elongation, image: an elongated object is distorted and appears longer on an x-ray image than it is clinically. Vertical underangulation of the PID or a physical curving (i.e. bending) a PSP plate when it is positioned intraorally will cause image elongation.

Embedded tooth: an unerupted tooth that is not prevented from normal eruption by an obstruction.

Erosion: the pathologic wearing down of tooth structure by chemical means.

Erythema: a superficial reddening of the skin.

Erythema dose: the radiation dose required to produce a redness of the skin. It generally occurs after exposure to 250 centisieverts (cSv) of radiation that is delivered in a relatively short span of 14 days. For comparison purposes, exposure doses from dental imaging are typically in microsieverts (mSv).

Evaginated crown: an abnormal protuberance on a crown.

Exostosis (pl exostoses): a benign self-limiting production of new bone that protrudes from the surface of an existing bone (e.g. osteoma, torus).

Exposure time: the duration of radiation generation. Modern intraoral x-ray units have exposure settings ranging from hundredths of a second to multiple seconds in length.

Extraoral: located outside of the mouth.

Extraoral image: an image acquired when the image receptor is positioned outside of the

patient's mouth. Extraoral dental projections include panoramic, cephalometric and CBCT imaging.

Fetal badge: a radiation dosimeter for a pregnant worker used to monitor radiation dose to the fetus over the term of the pregnancy.

Field of view (FOV): regarding CBCT images, it refers to the collimated area that is being imaged.

Film, non-screen: all intraoral dental x-ray film is classified as *non-screen film* because it does not use an *intensifying screen*. If an incoming x-ray photon collides with one of the silver halide crystals in the film emulsion, then it will precipitate out as a silver atom during chemical processing. As a result, a non-screen film requires more radiation to produce an image compared to screen film but it will produce a comparatively higher resolution image. Synonym: direct exposure film.

Film, screen: all extraoral dental x-ray film types are categorized as *screen film*. Unlike non-screen film, this category of film must be manually loaded into a film cassette. Each cassette will contain a pair of intensifying screens that surround the film on both the front and back sides. An intensifying screen contains rare earth minerals and phosphor materials that convert incoming x-ray photons into visible light. The emitted light from the screen exposes multiple silver halide crystals in the film's emulsion. Consequently there is a reduction in the total number of x-ray photons required to produce an image but it also lowers the image resolution compared to non-screen film images. Synonym: indirect exposure film.

Film, x-ray: this is composed of a polyester base that is coated with an emulsion. The film emulsion is a mixture of silver halide crystals embedded within a gelatin base. A developed piece of x-ray film is referred to as a *radiograph*. The dental radiographs are typically inserted into a film mount to secure them and then they are viewed on a lighted *view box* or a *light box*.

For many years, x-ray film was the standard for recording dental images. Today, it has largely been replaced by digital imaging receptors.

Filter, x-ray: typically a 1.5–2.5 mm thick sheet of aluminum built into all dental x-ray tubeheads. It is used to absorb (i.e. block) low energy x-ray photons before they can exit the x-ray unit. Filtering removes low energy x-ray photons that will not be able to penetrate through a patient's tissues to expose the image receptor. These low energy x-ray photons are of no benefit to either the operator or patient.

Flat panel detector: a solid-state digital x-ray receptor commonly used in CBCT x-ray units. It may be either an *indirect* or a *direct receptor*.

Floating tooth: a root of a tooth that is completely surrounded by a radiolucent area. It exhibits a complete absence of both the lamina dura and the immediate surrounding alveolar bone.

Focal spot: the tungsten target of the anode inside an x-ray tube. It is the location where the accelerated electrons emanating from the cathode are directed. The focal spot is where x-ray photons are generated.

Focal trough: an invisible three-dimensional zone specific for each extraoral x-ray unit. Laser lights on the x-ray unit are typically used to assist the operator in positioning the patient. Alignment of the patient by the operator in the focal trough will most accurately reproduce structures such as the mandible and maxilla. An operator's failure to properly position the patient in the focal trough will result in distortion and an overall decrease in the quality of the image.

Fog, image: an undesirable darkening of an image that produces a loss of image contrast. It is typically caused by scatter radiation. Fogging produced by *light leakage* is unique to x-ray film; light from an external light source exposes the unprocessed film.

Foreign body: any object or material that is not normal for the area in which it is located.

Foreshortened, image: vertical overangulation of an x-ray beam will distort the image of an object, making the object appear shorter on a dental image than its true length.

Frenulum: a small fold of mucous membrane that secures or restricts the movement of a mobile structure (e.g. tongue, lip). Synonym: frenum.

Full mouth series (FMS or FMX): a series of intraoral periapical and bitewing images that show all of the edentulous and edentulous areas of the mouth. The total number of images in an FMX is variable; it depends upon the size of the mandible and the maxilla, the number of teeth, etc. A typical FMX requires 15–20 individual images. Synonym: complete mouth series (CMX).

Generalized bone lesion: a lesion involving an entire bony structure.

Genetic effects of radiation: the effects of radiation on the *germ cells*. Changes produced in the genes and chromosomes of the germ cells may affect future offspring of the exposed individuals.

Germ cells: the oocytes and the spermatocytes. They are also sometimes referred to as *genetic cells* or *reproductive cells*. These cell types differ from *somatic cells* which comprise all of the other tissue cell types. The effects of radiation differ between germ and somatic cells.

Gestalt: can simply be described as seeing the whole picture.

Ghost image: a faint radiopaque shadow of an object or structure superimposed over normal anatomic structures on the opposite side of the patient and found on extraoral images. Ghost images are magnified, somewhat blurred and less radiopaque than the object itself. It will always occur on the contralateral side and slightly superior to the object of origin. Synonym: ghost shadow.

Gray (Gy): this unit quantifies the energy absorbed by a given material. The SI unit is called the *gray*. One gray is equivalent to 100 rad.

Ground glass appearance: a very fine bone trabecular pattern resulting in a diffuse radiopacity that visually resembles *ground glass* material; it often is associated with the late stage of fibrous dysplasia. (See Fig. X3.)

Hair-on-end appearance: fine, uniformly arranged spicules of bone starting from the inner table of the cranial vault and extending beyond the outer surface up to a couple of centimeters. The outer cortical plate is absent.

Half value layer (HVL): the thickness of material required to reduce the intensity of an x-ray beam by 50%. It is used to measure the penetrating ability or quality of an x-ray beam.

Hamular process: a short, hook-like process extending inferiorly from the medial pterygoid plate. It may be observed on intraoral images of the maxillary tuberosity as a thin, radiopaque projection angled down and posteriorly from the medial pterygoid plate. The gap between the hamular process and the maxillary tuberosity is referred to as the hamular notch.

Hertz (Hz): the SI unit of electrical frequency. It is equal to one cycle per second. In the United States, household electricity has a frequency of 60 cycles per second or 60 Hz, while in European countries the electrical frequency is 50 Hz.

HIPAA (Health Information Portability and Accountability Act): enacted by the US Congress in 1996 to address the use and disclosure of individuals' personal health information and to protect health insurance coverage for workers and families when they change or lose jobs.

Hittorf–Crookes tube: see Crookes–Hittorf tube.

Honeycomb appearance: a trabecular pattern having multiple, uniform, typically 2–5 mm oval or round radiolucent compartments in bone. Synonym: polycystic (Fig. X5).

Horizontal bone loss: the horizontal destruction of the crestal alveolar bone adjacent to the root surface of two or more teeth.

Hydroxyapatite: the main mineral of which tooth enamel and dentin are composed. Synonym: hydroxylapatite.

Hypercementosis: the deposition of excess cementum along a root surface; it often produces a bulbous radiographic appearance of the root.

Hypocalcified enamel: the correct total amount of enamel but the enamel is undercalcified.

Hypoplastic enamel: enamel that has a normal image density, but its thickness has been reduced.

Iatrogenic: something that was inadvertently caused by a medical or dental procedure.

Indirect digital imaging: the conversion of a latent image into a visible image. Initially a PSP plate directly captures and stores an x-ray image as a latent image. This latent image is then *indirectly* converted into a digital image with the use of a special laser scanner. This differs from a solid-state receptor, which directly sends the image to a computer without the need of a scanner.

Image enhancement: the process within a software program whereby the appearance of a digital image is altered. This is typically modified with the brightness, contrast, filtering and colorization controls.

Impaction: a tooth that is physically obstructed and unable to fully erupt into the dental arch.

Impaction, bony: an impacted tooth that is obstructed by both bone and soft tissue.

Impaction, dental: an impacted tooth that is obstructed by a barrier such as a neighboring tooth.

Incipient caries: a caries less than halfway through the enamel; from the meaning of incipient being something that is in an early stage of development.

Intensifying screen: a screen composed of rare earth materials that multiply the effect of incoming x-ray photons and thereby reduce the radiation exposure to the patient. The primary disadvantage of using an intensifying screen is that it reduces the overall resolution of the final radiographic image. Extraoral x-ray film is sandwiched between two intensifying screens that cover the front and back of the film within a light-tight cassette.

Invagination of a crown: an inward fold or cleavage of a crown.

Inverse square law: this law states that the intensity of radiation at a given point is inversely proportional to the mathematical square of the distance from the source of radiation. Simply stated, this means that if you double the distance of the source of radiation to the receptor, only one-quarter of the radiation will reach the receptor. With increasing distance the x-ray beam diverges covering a much larger field. To acquire the same amount of exposure at double the distance, the exposure time would need to be quadrupled.

Ionizing radiation: any type of electromagnetic radiation that has sufficient energy to knock an electron out of its atomic orbit. The process of producing an ion by removing an electron is referred to as *ionization*. Although it is not sharply demarcated, ionizing forms of radiation include shorter wavelength ultraviolet radiation, x radiation and gamma radiation.

Isometry: the mathematical rule of isometry states that two triangles are equal when they share a common side. As it applies to the bisecting angle intraoral technique, the bisector is the common side.

Kerma, air (kinetic energy released per unit mass): the sum of the initial kinetic energies of all the charged particles liberated by indirectly ionizing radiation per unit mass of a specified material.

Kilovolt (kV): 1 kV is 1000 V; 60–80 kV is the standard range for intraoral exposures. Kilovoltage represents the potential difference between the cathode and anode in the x-ray tube. The "p" in kVp indicates the maximum or peak voltage applied across an x-ray tube.

Kinetic energy: the energy of a mass in motion. In an x-ray tube, electrons accelerate from the cathode to the anode when a high voltage is applied. A very small percentage of that kinetic energy is converted into x-ray photons.

Lace-like appearance: a bone pattern that resembles fine threads. Synonyms: net, regular network.

Lagniappe: means something extra.

Lamina dura: the radiopaque line forming the outline of the tooth socket in the alveolar bone.

Latent image: a recorded image produced after exposure to radiation that cannot be visualized until it is digitally or chemically processed. A PSP plate stores a latent image until it is scanned. A dental x-ray film requires chemical processing.

Latent period: the period of time between exposure to radiation and the onset of symptoms.

Lateral cephalograph: a head profile projection that reveals osseous structures and soft tissue outline of the face. It is typically used in orthodontics for assessing facial growth and development. Alternatively, a lateral skull image does not use a cephalostat nor does it show the soft tissue outline in the image.

Law of Bergonie and Tribondeau: a fundamental law of radiation biology formulated in 1906 by Jean Bergonie, a French radiologist, and Louis Tribondeau, a French physician. The law states that the faster a cell replicates, the more sensitive it will be to radiation, and the more specialized a cell type is, the less sensitive it will be to the effects of radiation. Only two human cell types are currently known to contradict this law. These are the *lymphocytes* and the *oocytes*. Both of these cell types are specialized and they are very sensitive to radiation.

Line pairs per millimeter (lp/mm): a physical line plus the space adjacent to it is called a *line pair*. The number of line pairs distinguishable within a space of 1 mm is used as a measurement of x-ray image resolution. The higher the number of line pairs per millimeter visible, the greater is the resolution of the image. High resolution is useful for the detection of caries, a hairline tooth or bone fractures, etc.

Lingual foramen: is a tiny opening located on the lingual aspect of midline of the mandible. The lingual artery passes through it. The genial tubercles are frequently seen surrounding it on anterior periapical images.

Long PID: a PID (position indicating device) is considered long when the distance from the source of radiation (i.e. focal spot) to the position of the intraoral receptor is 30 cm or greater; a long PID is required when performing the paralleling technique. Synonym: long cone.

Lymphocyte: a specialized white blood cell in the immune system.

Mach band effect: an optical illusion that exaggerates the contrast along the borders of objects with differing densities. This can occur along the border of dentin and enamel. An illusionary radiolucent line may be produced which may lead to an erroneous diagnosis of a fracture or caries where none exist.

Magnetic resonance imaging (MRI): MRI was invented by Paul Lauterbur together with Sir Peter Mansfield who developed the mathematical technique for reconstructing images in 1971. MRI is non-invasive and uses non-ionizing radiation, unlike ionizing radiation which is typically used for conventional advanced dental imaging techniques such as CBCT. MRI is best for imaging the soft tissues. In dentistry, its usefulness is limited to soft tissue pathology, the study of the cartilaginous disk of the temporomandibular joint and for cosmetic oral and maxillofacial surgery. Disadvantages for dentistry are the high cost of the imaging procedure, long scan times and imaging artifacts from metallic restorations (e.g. amalgams, gold crowns). In addition, any ferromagnetic objects such as aneurysm clips may undergo movement as a

result of the strong magnetic field and can result in unexpected injury to a patient. For this procedure, the patient is positioned in a large magnet. The magnetic field generated temporarily results in the realignment and orientation of the protons, particularly hydrogen, which comprises approximately 70% of the patient's body. A radio wave signal is aimed at the patient and it is absorbed by some of the hydrogen nuclei. The radio signal is then turned off, the absorbed energy is released from the nuclei and it is detected as a signal by a coil in the scanner. A computer program then constructs the soft tissue images.

Malocclusion: see Occlusion.

Maximum occupational dose: government regulates the maximum amount of occupational radiation exposure that a worker can receive in a designated period of time. A radiation dosimeter will record the wearer's total exposure to radiation. Occupational workers are permitted to receive up to 5 centisieverts (cSv) in any one year.

Maximum permissible dose (MPD): as defined by the *International Commission on Radiation Protection* (ICRP), MPD is the permissible dose an individual can either accumulate over a long period of time or receive from a single exposure that carries a negligible probability of severe somatic or germ cell injuries.

Mid-sagittal: an imaginary line that anteroposteriorly divides the body along the midline. Synonym: mid-sagittal plane.

Milliampere (mA): 1 mA is one one-thousandth of an ampere.

Milliampere second (mAs): refers to the quantity of radiation produced. It is calculated by the milliampere setting and the selected exposure time. It affects image density.

Moth-eaten appearance: a poorly defined radiolucent area of bone composed of coalescing, multiple, irregular-shaped radiolucencies ranging in size from a few millimeters to several centimeters. These radiolucencies show some opacification, indicating only a partial loss of trabeculae within them.

Mulberry molar: describes a hypoplasia of enamel of one or more permanent maxillary or mandibular first molars. There is a characteristic constriction of the cusps and the occlusal surface that gives a crown a "pinched" appearance. The mulberry molar appears normal on x-ray images, except that it often has short roots. There is no racial or sexual predilection. Synonyms: Moon's molars and Fournier molars.

Multilocular appearance: an irregular pattern of multiple, non-uniform radiolucent compartments on bone. Synonym: polycystic. (See Fig. X1.)

Multiplanar reconstruction (MPR): the raw data accumulated from a CBCT scan that is converted by a software program into sagittal, coronal and axial planar images.

Nanometer (nm): a unit of spatial measurement that is one billionth of a meter.

Nasal septum: the dividing wall composed of bone and cartilage that runs down the center of the nasal fossa. (See Fig. U4.)

Nasion: the middle point of the junction of the frontal and two nasal bones. Superficially, it is the midpoint between the patient's eyes. It is a commonly used cephalometric landmark for orthodontic evaluation.

Nasolacrimal canal: contains the nasolacrimal duct and opens beneath the inferior nasal concha. On periapical images, it may occasionally be observed as a small ovoid radiolucency located superior to the apex of the cuspid.

Negative vertical angulation: the direction of the PID when it originates from below the occlusal plane and it is directed upwards.

Nutrient canals: thin channels within bone carrying nerve and blood vessels. They will appear on x-ray images as thin radiolucent lines often in the mandibular anterior region. Synonym: neurovascular canals.

Occlusal plane: an imaginary plane formed by the occlusal surfaces of the maxillary and mandibular teeth when the jaws are closed together.

Occlusal image: a topographic projection of either the maxilla or mandible utilizing either the bisecting angle or cross-sectional technique; useful for localization of impactions, fractures, root tips, and foreign bodies.

Occlusion, class I: the mesiobuccal cusp of the maxillary first molar aligns with the buccal groove of the mandibular first molar.

Occlusion, class II: the buccal groove of the mandibular first molar is distally positioned when in occlusion with the mesio-buccal cusp of the maxillary first molar.

Occlusion, class III: the buccal groove of the mandibular first molar is mesially positioned when in occlusion with the mesio-buccal cusp of the maxillary first molar.

Onion peel appearance thin layers of calcified bone tissue located adjacent and parallel to the outer surface of the cortical plate. Synonyms: layered, laminated.

Onlay restoration: an indirect restoration that is fabricated extraorally. It is fabricated for a tooth that does not require a full crown and when a conventional restoration may be structurally unsound. An onlay typically incorporates a tooth cusp.

Oocyte: an immature female reproductive cell prior to fertilization.

Osteonecrosis: bone degeneration as a result of decreased blood flow. A deficiency of blood causes the bone to degenerate faster than the body can regenerate new bone. Synonyms: avascular necrosis, aseptic necrosis, ischemic necrosis.

Osteoradionecrosis of the jaws: the administration of high therapeutic doses of ionizing radiation for oral cancer (over 50 Gy) may result in irreversible hypovascular bone. Reduction in bone vascularity causes it to become more susceptible to infection and traumatic injury. The ultimate result is bone degenerating faster than the body can regenerate new bone. The mandible is more often affected than the maxilla. Osteoradionecrosis appears similar to osteomyelitis on x-ray images.

Overexposure, image: an x-ray image that overall appears too dark. Contributing factors may include any or all of the following: high kilovoltage, high milliamperage or long exposure time setting. X-ray film can be excessively dark from exposure to external light sources prior to processing.

Palatoglossal air space: the gap between the dorsal surface of the tongue and the palate. It may appear as a crescent-shaped radiolucent band across a panoramic image.

Panoramic image: an unobstructed two-dimensional extraoral view of the entire mouth in a single image. It captures all of the teeth, maxilla, mandible and surrounding structures. Synonym: pantomogram.

Panorex®: the commercial name for an early model of a panoramic unit (circa 1967) sold by the S. S. White Division of the Pennwalt Corp., Philadelphia, PA.

Paralleling technique: an intraoral technique where the long axis of the tooth and the receptor are positioned parallel to one another and the x-ray beam is aimed perpendicular to both of them. This maximizes the accuracy of the projected image and thus minimizes distortion.

Paresthesia: a transient or chronic sensation known as a *pins and needles tingling* of a person's skin. In dentistry, it typically arises from damage to the inferior alveolar nerve.

Particulate radiation: this is composed of atomic or subatomic particles having both mass and energy. Particulate radiation includes alpha particles, beta particles and neutrons.

Penumbra: the blurriness or area of unsharpness found along the edge of an x-ray image. Multiple factors can affect image unsharpness, including focal spot size, motion, tube–receptor distance and tube–object distance.

Periapical: refers to the region around the root tip (apex) of a tooth.

Periapical image: an intraoral image that shows one or more teeth in their entirety. In edentulous regions, a periapical image is useful for visualizing root tips, impactions and foreign bodies.

Periapical lesion: active or inactive pathology located at the apex of a tooth. It may be either a radiopaque or a radiolucent lesion.

Periapical scar: an unresolved periapical radiolucency associated with an endodontically treated tooth. It may be a periapical lesion that healed with fibrous tissue in lieu of mature bone.

Pericoronal: refers to the region around the crown of a tooth.

Pericoronitis: refers to the inflammation of the soft tissues surrounding the crown of a partially erupted tooth.

Periodontal ligament space (PDL space): the radiolucent gap (i.e. space) between the lamina dura and the root surface on an x-ray image. The PDL space may appear to be absent simply because the operator positioned the PID at an oblique angle to the buccal surface of the tooth. It is important to be aware that actual widening or loss of the PDL space may be an indicator of pathology.

Personal protection equipment (PPE): refers to the universal infection control guidelines as mandated in the United States by the Occupational Safety and Health Administration (OSHA). All dental personnel directly involved with patient care must wear protective clothing. Disposable or non-disposable gowns must be long-sleeved, at least three-quarter in length and have a closed collar. In addition, disposable protective gloves should always be worn by the operator during receptor and tubehead placement to minimize risks to both the operator and the patient. For x-ray imaging procedures, aerosols are not generated but exposure to bodily fluids is still unavoidable. Consequently, operators may wish to wear protective eyewear and a mask or face-shield. Image receptors must be covered with disposable plastic non-permeable wraps. Computer components (i.e. keyboard and mouse) and x-ray equipment (i.e. tubehead and control panel) should be protected with surface barriers that are changed after each patient. If barriers are not used, equipment that has come into contact with the operator's gloved hands should be cleaned and then disinfected after each patient use.

Phleboliths: typically are small, round calcifications located within venous structures, and are often associated with hemangiomas. (See Fig. X4.)

Photon: a packet of energy that has no mass. It is ascribed to electromagnetic radiation, which includes radio waves, visible light, x rays, gamma rays, etc.

Photostimulable phosphor plate (PSP plate): is a polyester base material coated with a halide emulsion. It stores the energy from incoming x-ray photons as a latent image. The latent image is then converted into visual image by a laser scanner. The PSP plate can be reused after erasure of the image, disinfection and repackaging. (See Indirect digital imaging.)

PID (position indicating device): the open-end extension off the x-ray tubehead through which x rays are directed. The shape of the PID may either be round or rectangular. Synonym: BID (beam indicating device).

Pixel: the smallest, basic component of a digital image that can be processed.

Pneumatization: the development of air cells (aka cavities) within a bone.

Positive vertical angulation: the direction of the PID when it originates from above the occlusal plane and it is directed downwards.

Primary radiation: the beam of radiation that directly exits the PID of an x-ray tubehead.

Processor, film: a device that is used to turn a latent x-ray image on a piece of x-ray film into a visible image with the use of chemical solutions. An *automatic film processor* is a machine that mechanically moves each film(s) through multiple chemical solutions to produce a visible image. The processed film is called a radiograph. *Manual film processing* involves an operator manually hand dipping the x-ray film(s) in different chemical solutions to produce a final radiograph.

Proprietor: the owner of a business.

Punched out appearance: one or more well-defined round or oval-shaped radiolucencies ranging in diameter from 1 cm to several centimeters. These radiolucencies show no opacification, such as trabeculae, within them.

Quality assurance: the regular monitoring of x-ray equipment to ensure that proper standards of quality are being met. The objective is to achieve optimum diagnostic images and the elimination of unnecessary radiation exposure to patients, occupational workers and the general public.

Quality of the x-ray beam: refers to the mean energy or penetrating ability of the x-ray photons. It is affected by the kilovoltage setting of the x-ray unit. It is characterized by its *half value layer*.

Quantity of the x-ray beam: refers to the total number of x-ray photons generated during an exposure. It is affected by the milliamperage, time and kilovoltage settings of the x-ray unit.

Radiation, natural background: see Background radiation.

Radiation absorbed dose (rad): the traditional unit for quantifying the energy absorbed by a given material. The SI unit for rad is called the *gray* (Gy). The conversion is 1 Gy equals 100 rad.

Radiation biology: the study of the effects of ionizing radiation on living things.

Radiation caries: an indirect effect of therapeutic irradiation. Radiotherapy for the treatment of oral cancer may result in the loss of function of the salivary glands. Reduced salivary flow places the individual in a higher risk category for dental caries. Radiotherapy may incapacitate the individual and limit their ability to maintain their oral hygiene adequately.

Radioactivity: the property of some unstable elements to spontaneously emit radiation. This may include alpha particles, beta particles and gamma rays.

Radiograph: a term originally used to apply to a visible image on a processed piece of x-ray film. The term radiograph is still used to describe digital x-ray images. Synonym: x-ray image.

Radiolucent: describes the penetrability of x-ray photons through an object to produce the darker colored regions on a radiograph.

Radiopaque: describes the impenetrability of x-ray photons through an object to produce the lighter colored regions on a radiograph.

Rectangular PID: a rectangular-shaped x-ray beam recommended by the National Council on Radiation Protection and Measurements for reducing the volumetric area of exposure to the patient compared to a conventional round PID. Synonym: rectangular collimator.

Rectification: the conversion of alternating current to direct current. *Self-rectification* is the property of an x-ray tube to restrict the flow of electricity to only one direction (i.e. from the cathode to the anode).

Residual cyst: a chronic cyst resulting from the incomplete removal of the original cyst.

Resolution, image: a measure of how closely two objects can be placed side by side and still be distinguishable as separate objects. Resolution of x-ray images is defined by the number of line pairs per millimeter that are discernible.

Resolution, spatial: refers to the number of pixels used in digital image construction.

Resorption, root: (1) *Smooth root resorption*: the root will appear shortened or blunted, but its surface is relatively smooth and it is surrounded by a distinct periodontal ligament space. (2) *Rough root resorption*: the root will appear with an irregular surface, with the periodontal ligament space either widened or non-existent. (3) *Internal resorption*: destruction of the dentin from the pulp chamber outwards creates a round or oval radiolucent area associated with the pulp. If it progresses far enough, it will reach the external surface of the root.

Roentgen (R): a measure of ionization produced in air by x rays or gamma rays. It was named after the discoverer of x rays, Professor Wilhelm Röntgen. Roentgen units have been replaced with the SI unit, coulombs per kilogram. One roentgen equals 258 µC/kg.

Roentgen equivalent man (rem): the traditional unit used to compare the biologic effects of different types of radiation on a tissue or organ. The SI unit for rem is called the *sievert* (Sv). The conversion is 1 Sv equals 100 rem.

Ruhmkorff coil: a type of transformer used to produce high voltages from low voltage direct current. It was originally used in conjunction with a Crookes–Hittorf tube to generate x rays.

Sagittal plane: the vertical plane that runs parallel to the median.

Scalloped appearance: a well-defined, undulating border with the indentations being of similar size.

Scanner, PSP plate: PSP plates must pass through a specialized laser scanner that reads and digitizes the acquired images. The processed images can then be viewed on a computer monitor.

Scatter radiation: the deviation of x-ray photons from their original path upon interaction with matter.

Sclerosis of bone: an ill-defined radiopaque area characterized by: (i) a reduction in the size of the trabecular spaces; (ii) an increase in the number of trabeculae and an increase in the opacity of the involved bone; and (iii) a variable, size ranging from millimeters to several centimeters. Synonyms: sclerosing osteitis, condensing osteitis, bone sclerosis.

Scoliosis: an abnormal curving of the spine.

Scout image: a preliminary CBCT image taken prior to the actual scan. Synonym: preview image.

Secondary radiation: a weaker form of x radiation produced after the incoming x rays interact with matter.

Septum, osseous (pl septae): a bony wall that subdivides a larger space.

Sharpness: the ability of the imaging receptor to define the edge of an object.

Short PID: a PID (position indicating device) is considered short when the distance from the source of radiation (i.e. focal spot) to the placement of the intraoral receptor is no more than 20 cm. Synonym: short cone.

Sievert (Sv): compares the biologic effects of different types of radiation on a tissue or organ. The SI unit is a sievert and replaces the traditional unit *rem*. One sievert is equivalent to 100 rem.

Sinus lift: a surgical bone augmentation procedure in the maxillary sinus to allow the placement of posterior implants when the maxillary alveolar ridge height is insufficient.

SLOB rule (same–lingual, opposite–buccal): an intraoral technique used to localize objects from a bucco-lingual perspective by exposing two images using different angulations. Objects that are on the lingual side will not appear to move, while objects towards the buccal side will shift in an opposite direction from the movement of the PID.

Soap bubble appearance: a grape-like cluster of circular compartments of variable size. Synonyms: multiloculated, polycystic. (See Fig. X1.)

Somatic cells: includes all of the tissue cell types in the body with the exception of the two germ cells, the *oocytes* and *spermatocytes*.

Somatic effects: the deleterious effects of radiation observed in the exposed individual only. The radiated individual's future offspring will not be affected if the germ cells were not affected by the radiation.

Sterilize: a mechanism for destroying all living microorganisms.

Stochastic effects: refers to the random biologic effects of radiation without a requirement to surpass a threshold exposure dose level. The probability of occurrence is proportional to the dose but the severity of the effect is independent of it. A primary stochastic effect is cancer. (See Deterministic effects.)

Submerged teeth: deciduous teeth that have undergone a degree of root resorption and have become ankylosed to the bone.

Sunburst appearance: description of fine or coarse spicules of bone that radiate perpendicularly from the cortical plate. The spicules may be few in number or form a continuous palisade with their length ranging from a few millimeters to a couple of centimeters. Synonyms: starburst, sunray. (See Fig. X7.)

Supernumerary tooth: the presence of an extra tooth in excess of the normal complement of teeth. A supernumerary tooth can be well-formed or misshaped.

Taurodont: a tooth with a large body and pulp chamber, very little root formation and an overall tooth size that is normal.

Threshold dose: the minimum exposure dose when a measurable effect will manifest itself.

Thyroid collar: additional shielding wrapped around the patient's neck to protect the thyroid gland from x-ray exposure.

Tomography: a technique for imaging a single plane of a three-dimensional object by blurring out structures both in front and behind the area of interest.

Tomogram: a thin sectional x-ray image of an object that is acquired with a tomographic x-ray unit.

Torus: a self-limiting bony growth typically located in the mandible near the bicuspids above the mylohyoid ridge and/or in the midline of the hardplate (PL tori).

Transformer: a device used to either increase or decrease voltage. A *step-down transformer* reduces the incoming voltage to the cathode in the x-ray tube. A *step-up transformer* increases the voltage between the cathode and the anode of an x-ray tube.

Transposition: the eruption of a tooth in an abnormal position in the dental arch. Any tooth may be affected, but there is a predilection for the permanent maxillary cuspids and bicuspids. Synonyms: translocated teeth, displaced teeth.

Trismus: a spasm of the muscles of mastication that restricts mouth opening.

Tubehead, intraoral: the metal housing that contains the x-ray tube, step-up and step-down transformers, lead collimator, aluminum filter, insulating oil and seals and has an attached PID. An intraoral tubehead may be mobile, fixed or hand-held.

Tumefaction: the process of becoming swollen.

Umbra: the area of the x-ray image proper. (See Penumbra.)

Underexposure, image: an x-ray image that overall appears too light. Contributing factors may include any or all of the following: low kilovoltage, low millamperage or a short exposure time setting.

Unilocular: a radiolucency consisting of only one compartment or chamber. Synonym: unicystic. (See Fig. X2.)

Universal precautions: a set of procedural directives and guidelines published in 1987 by the US Centers for Disease Control and Prevention (CDC) to prevent parenteral, mucous membrane and non-intact skin exposures of healthcare workers to blood-borne pathogens. In 1991, the Occupational Safety and Health Administration (OSHA) imposed requirements on employers of healthcare workers, including engineering controls, provision of protective barrier devices, standardized labeling of biohazards, mandatory training of employees in universal precautions, management of accidental parenteral exposure incidents and availability to employees of immunization against hepatitis B.

Vertical bone loss: the destruction of the crestal alveolar bone adjacent to the root surface of two or more teeth resulting in an angular surface.

View box: consists of an enclosure with a translucent surface through which light is transmitted. It is used to view processed dental x-ray films (i.e. radiographs). Synonyms: light box, illuminator.

Voxel: a three-dimensional space unlike the two-dimensional pixel. The term *voxel* is derived from a combination of *vol*ume and *el*ement.

Worm eaten appearance: description of bone composed of an irregular pattern of multiple radiolucent channels. The size of the channels can range up to several millimeters wide and up to several centimeters in length.

Xerostomia: is a dryness of the mouth as a result of a cessation of normal salivary secretion. It may be a side effect of medication or associated with systemic disorders, such as Sjogren's Syndrome. Patients receiving medical radiotherapy to treat oral cancer often experience loss of function of salivary glands.

X-ray source: the tungsten focal spot on the anode where x rays are generated.

X-ray unit: an apparatus that is used to generate x rays. Synonyms: x-ray machine, x-ray device, x-ray equipment.

Suggested Reading

Abaza N, EI-Khashab M, Kreutner Jr. A. (1971) Central myxoma of the mandible. *Oral Surg, Oral Med and Oral Pathol.* 31:465–71.

Abrahms AM, Kirby JW, Melrose RJ. (1974) Cementoblastoma. *Oral Surg, Oral Med and Oral Pathol.* 38:394–403.

Adekeye EO. (1980) Ameloblastoma of the jaws: a survey of 109 Nigerian patients. *J of Oral Surg.* 38:36–41.

Adekeye EO, Edwards MB, Goubran GF. (1978) Ameloblastic fibrosarcoma. *Oral Surg, Oral Med and Oral Pathol.* 46:254–9.

Adekeye EO, Edwards MB, Williams HK. (1984) Advanced central myxoma of the jaws in Nigeria. *Int J of Oral Surg.* 13:177–86.

Ai-Ru L, Zhen L, Jian S. (1982) Calcifying epithelial odontogenic tumors. *J of Oral Pathol.* 11:399–406.

Ajagbel A, Samuel I, Daramola JO. (1978) Giant cell tumor of the maxilla. *Oral Surg, Oral Med and Oral Pathol.* 46:759–64.

Akinosi JS, Olumide F, Ogunbiyi AJ. (1975) Retrosternal parathyroid adenomas manifesting in the form of a giant cell tumor of the mandible. *Oral Surg, Oral Med and Oral Pathol.* 3:724–33.

Alawi F. (2002) Benign fibro-osseous diseases of the maxillofacial bones. A review and differential diagnosis. *Am J Clin Pathol.* 118(Suppl):S50–70.

Allard RHB, van der Waal I, van der Kwast AM. (1981) Mucosal antral cysts. *Oral Surg, Oral Med and Oral Pathol.* 51:2–9.

Allard RHB, van der Waal I, van der Kwast AM. (1981) Nasopalatine duct cyst. *Int J of Oral Surg.* 10:447–61.

Alsufyani NA, Lam EW. (2011) Cemento-osseous dysplasia of the jaw bones: key radiographic features. *Dentomaxillofac Radiol.* 40:141–6.

Alsufyani NA, Lam EW. (2011) Osseous (cemento-osseous) dysplasia of the jaws: clinical and radiographic analysis. *J Can Dent Assoc.* 77:b70.

Altini M, Cohen M, (1982) The follicular primordial cyst – odontogenic keratocyst. *Int J Oral Surg.* 11:175–82.

Altini M, Shear M. (1992) The lateral periodontal cyst: an update. *J Oral Pathol Med.* 21:245–50.

American Dental Association. (2012) *Dental Radiographic Examinations: Recommendations for Patient Selection and Limiting Radiation Exposure.* ADA Council on Scientific Affairs, US Dept of Health and Human Services, Public Health Service, Food and Drug Administration.

American Dental Association Council on Scientific Affairs. (2006) The use of dental radiographs: update and recommendations. *J Am Dent Assoc.* 137:1304–12.

Angelopoulou E, Angelopoulos AP. (1990) Lateral periodontal cyst. Review of the literature and report of a case. *J Periodontol.* 61(2):126–31.

Angiero F, Moltrasio F, Cattoretti G, Valente MG. (2011) Clinical and histopathological profiles of primary or secondary osteosarcoma of the jaws. *Anticancer Res.* 31(12):4485–9.

Anneroth G, Hansen LS. (1982) Variations in keratinizing odontogenic cysts and tumors. *Oral Surg, Oral Med and Oral Pathol.* 53:546.

Anneroth G, Isacsson G, Sigurdsson A. (1975) Benign cementoblastoma (true cementoma). *Oral Surg, Oral Med and Oral Pathol.* 40:141–6.

Anneroth G, Johansson B. (1985) Peripheral ameloblastoma. *Int J of Oral Surg.* 11:295–9.

Ariji Y, Ariji E, Higuchi Y, Kubo S, Nakayama E, Kanda S. (1994) Florid cemento-osseous dysplasia. Radiographic study with special emphasis on computed tomography. *Oral Surg, Oral Med and Oral Pathol.* 78:391–6.

Arlen M, Tollefsen HR, Huvos AG, Marcove, RC. (1970) Chondrosarcoma of the head and neck. *Am J of Surg.* 120:456–61.

Arndt CAS. (2011) *Benign Tumors and Tumor-like Processes of Bone*, 19th edn. Saunders-Elsevier, Philadelphia.

Arnott DG. (1978) Cherubism – an initial unilateral presentation. *Br J of Oral Surg.* 16:38–45.

Astacio JN, Mendez JE. (1974) Benign cementoblastoma (true cementoma). *Oral Surg, Oral Med and Oral Pathol.* 38:95–9.

August M, Magennis P, Dewitt D. (1997) Osteogenic sarcoma of the jaws: factors which influence the prognosis. *Int J Oral Maxillofac Surg.* 26:198–204.

Austinj Jr. LT, Dahlin DC, Royer RQ. (1959) Giant-cell reparative granuloma and related conditions affecting the jawbones. *Oral Surg, Oral Med and Oral Pathol.* 12:1285–95.

Azzato N. (1957) Primary chondrosarcoma of the mandible. *Plastic and Reconstructive Surg.* 19:137–42.

Baker RD, D'Onofrio ED, Corio RL, Crawford BE, Terry BC. (1979) Squamous-cell carcinoma arising in a lateral periodontal cyst. *Oral Surg, Oral Med and Oral Pathol.* 47(6):495–9.

Barker BF, Jenson JL, Howell FV. (1974) Focal osteoporotic bone marrow defects of the jaws. *Oral Surg, Oral Med and Oral Pathol.* 38:404–13.

Barnes R. (1956) Aneurysmal bone cyst. *J of Bone and Joint Surg.* 38:301–11.

Barros RE, Dominguez FV, Cabrini RL. (1969) Myxoma of the jaws. *Oral Surg, Oral Med and Oral Pathol.* 27:225–37.

Basu MK, Matthews JB, Sear AJ, Browne, RM. (1984) Calcifying epithelial odotogenic tumour. *J of Oral Pathol.* 13:310–9.

Bataineh AB, al Qudah M. (1998) Treatment of mandibular odontogenic keratocysts. *Oral Surg Oral Med Oral Pathol Oral Radiol Endod.* 86(1):42–7.

Batcheldor GD, Giansanti JS, Hibbard ED, Waldron CA. (1973) Garre's osteomyelitis of the jaws. *J Am Dent Assoc.* 87:892–7.

Baty JM, Vogt EC. (1935) Bone changes of leukemia in children. *Am J of Roentgenol.* 34:310–3.

Beighton P, Horan F, Hamersma H. (1977) A review of the osteopetroses. *Postgraduate Med J.* 507–17.

Bell WH. (1959) Sclerosing osteomyelitis of the mandible and maxilla. *Oral Surg, Oral Med and Oral Pathol.* 12:391–401.

Bender IB. (1944) Bone changes in leukemia. *Am J of Ortho and Oral Surg.* 30:556–63.

Bender IB. (2003) Paget's disease. *J Endod.* 29:720–3.

Bennett JH, Thomas G, Evans AW, Speight PM. (2000) Osteosarcoma of the jaws: a 30-year retrospective review. *Oral Surg Oral Med Oral Pathol Oral Radiol Endod.* 90:323–33.

Berger A. (1947) Solitary central giant-cell tumor of the jawbones. *J of Oral Surg.* 5:154–66.

Berger A, Jaffe HL. (1953) Fibrous (fibro-osseous) dysplasia of the jawbones. *J of Oral Surg.* 11:3–17.

Bernier JL, Bhaskar SN. (1958) Aneurysmal bone cysts of the mandible. *Oral Surg, Oral Med and Oral Pathol.* 11:1018–28.

Bernstein HF, Lam RC, Pomije FW. (1958) Static bone cavities of the mandible: review of the literature and report of case. *J of Oral Surg.* 16:46–52.

Bernstein ML, Neal DC. (1985) Oral lesion in a patient with calcinosis and arthritis. *J of Oral Surg.* 14:8–14.

Bertelli A, Costa FQ, Miziara J. (1970) Metastatic tumors of the mandible. *Oral Surg, Oral Med and Oral Pathol.* 30:21–9.

Beylouni I, Farge P, Mazoyer JF, Coudert JL. (1998) Florid cemento-osseous dysplasia: report of a case documented with computed tomography and 3D imaging. *Oral Surg Oral Med Oral Pathol Oral Radiol Endod.* 85(6):707–11.

Beziat JL, Marcelino JP, Bascoulergue Y, Vitrey D. (1997) Central vascular malformation of the mandible: a case report. *J Oral Maxillofac Surg.* 55:415–9.

Bhaskar SN. (1968) Oral pathology in the dental office: survey of 2,575 biopsy specimens. *J of Am Dent Assoc.* 76:761–6.

Bhaskar SN. (1977) *Synopsis of Oral Pathology*. Mosby, St. Louis.

Bhoweer AL, Shirwatkar LG. (1975) Central hemangioma of mandible. *J of Oral Med.* 30:111–3.

Biorklund A, Elner A, Snorradottir M. (1979) Ameloblastoma of the maxilla: report of three cases. *J of Larynol and Otol.* 93:1105–13.

Black BK, Ackerman LV. (1950) Tumors of the parathyroid. *Cancer.* 3:415–31.

Bluestone LI. (1953) Malignant melanoma metastatic to the mandible. *Oral Surg, Oral Med and Oral Pathol.* 6:237–42.

Bodner L, Bar-Ziv J. (1996) Radiographic features of central giant cell granuloma of the jaws in children. *Pediatr Radiol.* 26:148–51.

Boston HC, Dahlin DC, Ivins JC, Cupps RE. (1974) Malignant lymphoma (so-called reticulum cell sarcoma) of bone. *Cancer.* 34:1131–7.

Bouckaert MM, Roubenheimer EJ, Jacobs FJ. (2000) Calcifying epithelial odontogenic tumor with intracranial extension: report of a case and review of literature. *Oral Surg Oral Med Oral Pathol Oral Radiol Endod.* 90:656–62.

Boyd RC. (1979) Aneurysmal bone cysts of the jaws. *Br J of Oral Surg.* 16:248–53.

Boysen ME, Olving JH, Vatne K, Koppang HS. (1979) Fibro-osseous lesions of the craniofacial bones. *J of Laryngol and Otol.* 93:793–7.

Brannon RB. (1976) The odontogenic keratocyst. *Oral Surg, Oral Med and Oral Pathol.* 42:54–71.

Brannon RB, Fowler CB. (2001) Benign fibro-osseous lesions: a review of current concepts. *Adv Anat Pathol.* 8(3):126–43.

Brannon RB, Fowler CB, Carpenter WM, Corio RL. (2002) Cementoblastoma: an innocuous neoplasm? A clinico-pathologic study of 44 cases and review of the literature with special emphasis on recurrence. *Oral Surg Oral Med Oral Pathol Oral Radiol Endod.* 93:311–20.

Bras JM, Donner R, van der Kwast AM, Snow GB, van der Waal I. (1980) Juxtacortical osteogenic sarcoma of the jaws. *Oral Surg, Oral Med and Oral Pathol.* 50:535–43.

Brodsky HR. (1934) Mandibular cavernous hemangioma. *Dental Digest.* 40:60–4.

Brødum N, Jensen VJ. (1991) Recurrence of keratocysts and decompression treatment. A long-term follow-up of forty-four cases. *Oral Surg, Oral Med and Oral Pathol.* 72(3):265–9.

Bruce KW, Royer RQ. (1952) Central myxoma of the maxilla. *Oral Surg, Oral Med and Oral Pathol.* 5:1277–81.

Bruce KW, Royer RQ. (1953) Multiple myeloma occurring in the jaws. *Oral Surg, Oral Med and Oral Pathol.* 6:729–44.

Brustein HC, Mautner RL. (1976) Osteogenesis imperfecta. *Oral Surg, Oral Med and Oral Pathol.* 42:42–52.

Buchner A. (1991) The central (intraosseous) calcifying odontogenic cyst: an analysis of 215 cases. *J Oral Maxillofac Surg.* 49:330–9.

Budnick SD. (1976) Compound and complex odontomas. *Oral Surg, Oral Med and Oral Pathol.* 42:511–5.

Bunel K, Sindet-Pedersen S. (1993) Central hemangioma of the mandible. *Oral Surg, Oral Med and Oral Pathol.* 75:565–70.

Burland JG. (1962) Cherubism: familial bilateral osseous dysplasia of the jaws. *Oral Surg, Oral Med and Oral Pathol.* 15:43–68.

Butt WP, Hollender L, Stener I. (1969). Mandibular erosion in tumours of the major salivary glands. *Acta Radiol.* 8:235–40.

Byrd DL, Kindrick RD, Dunsworth AR. (1973) Myxoma of the maxilla. *J of Oral Surg.* 31:123–6.

Cabrini RL, Barros RE, Albano H. (1970) Cysts of the jaws: a statistical analysis. *J of Oral Surg.* 28:485–9.

Caffey J, Williams JL. (1951) Familial fibrous swelling of the jaws. *Radiology.* 56:1–13.

Calman HI. (1952) Multiple myeloma. *Oral Surg, Oral Med and Oral Pathol.* 5:1302–11.

Campos PSF, Panella J, Crusoe'Rebello IM, Azevedo RA, Pena N, Cunha T. (2004) Mandibular ramus-related Stafne's bone cavity. *Dentomaxillofac Radiol.* 33:63–6.

Canalis RF, Smith GA, Konrad HR. (1976) Myxomas of the head and neck. *Arch of Otolaryngol.* 102:300–5.

Cangiano R, Mooney J, Stratigos GT. (1972) Osteopetrosis. *J of Oral Surg.* 30:217–22.

Cannon ML, Spiegel RE, Cooley RO. (1983) Hereditary fibrous dysplasia of the jaws (cherubism): report of a case. *J of Dent for Child.* July–August:292–5.

Caravolas JG, Pierce JM, Andrews JE, Nazif M. (1981) Mesenchymal chondrosarcoma of the mandible. *Oral Surg, Oral Med and Oral Pathol.* 52:478–4.

Carder HM, Hill JJ. (1966) Asymptomatic rhinolith: a brief review of the literature and case report. *Laryngoscope.* 3: 524–9.

Carlson ER, Marx RE. (2006) The ameloblastoma: primary, curative surgical management. *J Oral Maxillofac Surg.* 64(3):484–94.

Caron AS, Hajdu SI, Strong EW. (1971) Osteogenic sarcoma of the facial and cranial bones. *Am J of Surg.* 122:719–25.

Carr RF, Halperin V. (1968) Malignant ameloblastomas from 1953–1966. *Oral Surg, Oral Med and Oral Pathol.* 26:514–22.

Carter LC, Carney YL, Perez-Pudlewski D. (1996) Lateral periodontal cyst. Multifactorial analysis of a previously unreported series. *Oral Surg Oral Med Oral Pathol Oral Radiol Endod.* 81(2):210–6.

Carvalho Silva E, Carvalho Silva GC, Vieira TC. (2007) Cherubism: clinicoradiographic features, treatment, and long-term follow-up of 8 cases. *J Oral Maxillofac Surg.* 65(3):517–22.

Cash CD, Royer RQ. (1961) Metastatic tumors of the jaws. *Oral Surg, Oral Med and Oral Pathol.* 14:897–905.

Cataldo E, Meyer I. (1966) Solitary and multiple plasma cell tumors of the jaws and oral cavity. *Oral Surg, Oral Med and Oral Pathol.* 22:630–9.

Centers for Disease Control and Prevention. (2016) *Summary of Infection Prevention Practices in Dental Settings: Basic Expectations for Safe Care.* Centers for Disease Control and Prevention, US Department of Health and Human Services, Atlanta, GA.

Chadwick JW, Alsufyani NA, Lam EW. (2011) The clinical and radiographic features of solitary and cemento-osseous dysplasia-associated simple bone cysts. *Dentomaxillofac Radiol.* 40(4):230–5.

Chaudhry AP, Hayes PA, Gorlin RJ. (1958) Hyperparathyroidism involving the mandible. *J of Oral Surg.* 16:247–51.

Chaudhry AP, Robinovitch MR, Mitchell DF, Vickers RA. (1961) Chondrogenic tumors of the jaws. *Am J of Surg.* 102:403–10.

Chaudhry AP, Spink JH, Gorlin RJ. (1958) Periapical fibrous dysplasia. *J of Oral Surg.* 11:483–8.

Chaudhry AP, Vickers RA, Gorlin RJ. (1961) Intraoral minor salivary gland tumors. *Oral Surg, Oral Med and Oral Pathol.* 14:1194–223.

Chaudhuri P. (1978) Ameloblastoma. *J of Laryngol and Otol.* 92:457–65.

Chehade A, Daley TD, Wysocki GP, Miller AS. (1994) Peripheral odontogenic keratocyst. *Oral Surg, Oral Med and Oral Pathol.* 77(5):494–7.

Cheng NC, Lai DM, Hsie MH, Liao SL, Chen YB. (2006) Intraosseous hemangiomas of the facial bone. *Plast Reconstr Surg.* 117(7):2366–72.

Cherrick HM, King Jr. OH, Lucatorto FM, Suggs DM. (1974) Benign cementoma. *Oral Surg, Oral Med and Oral Pathol.* 37:54–63.

Chindia ML. (2001) Osteosarcoma of the jaw bones. *Oral Oncol.* 37(7):545–7.

Cho BH, Jung YH, Nah KS. (2007) The prevalence, clinical and radiographic characteristics of cemento-osseous dysplasia in Korea. *Korean J Oral Maxillofac Radiol.* 37:185–9.

Chow HT. (1998) Odontogenic keratocyst: a clinical experience in Singapore. *Oral Surg Oral Med Oral Pathol Oral Radiol Endod.* 86(5):573–7.

Christensen Jr. RE. (1982) Mesenchymal chondrosarcoma jaws. *Oral Surg, Oral Med and Oral Pathol.* 54:197–206.

Christensen Jr. RE, Propper RH. (1982) Intraosseous mandibular cyst with sebaceous differentiation. *Oral Surg, Oral Med and Oral Pathol.* 53:591–5.

Christensen RW. (1956) Complex composite odontoma involving the maxilla and maxillary sinus. *Oral Surg, Oral Med and Oral Pathol.* 9:1156–9.

Chuong R, Donoff R, Guralnick W. (1982) The odontogenic keratocyst. *J of Oral Surg.* 40:797–803.

Cicconetti A, Tallarico M, Bartoli A, Ripari A, Maggiani F. (2004) Calcifying epithelial odontogenic (Pindborg) tumor: a clinical case. *Minerva Stomatol.* 53:379–87.

Ciola B. (1981) Oral radiographic manifestations of a prostatic carcinoma. *Oral Surg, Oral Med and Oral Pathol.* 52:105–8.

Ciola B, Catema DL, Khang PH. (1975) Radiographic manifestations of a chronic apical rarefying osteitis with an unusual fistulous tract. *Oral Surg, Oral Med and Oral Pathol.* 39:654–7.

Ciola B, Yesner R. (1977) Radiographic manifestations of a lung carcinoma with metastases to the anterior maxilla. *Oral Surg, Oral Med and Oral Pathol.* 44:811–5.

Clausen F, Poulsen H. (1963) Metastatic carcinoma to the jaws. *Acta Path et Micro Scand.* 7:361–74.

Clemett A, Williams JH. (1963) The familial occurrence of infantile cortical hyperostosis. *Radiology.* 80:409–16.

Cline RE, Stenger TG. (1977) Histiocytic lymphoma (reticulum-cell sarcoma). *Oral Surg, Oral Med and Oral Pathol.* 43:422–35.

Cohen J. (1951) Osteopetrosis. *J of Bone and Joint Surg.* 33A:923–37.

Cohen M. (1984) Hemorrhagic (traumatic) cyst of the mandible associated with a retained root apex. *Oral Surg, Oral Med and Oral Pathol.* 57:26–7.

Cohen MA, Mendelsohn DB, Hertzanu Y. (1984) Chondrosarcoma of the maxilla. *Int J of Oral Surg.* 13:528–31.

Cohen S, Becker GL. (1976) Origin, diagnosis and treatment of the dental manifestations of vitamin D resistant rickets. *J of Am Dent Assoc.* 92:120–9.

Conley J, Stout AP, Healey WV. (1967) Clinicopathologic analysis of eighty-four patients with an original diagnosis of fibrosarcoma of the head and neck. *Am J of Surg.* 114:564–9.

Cook HP. (1961) Oral lymphomas. *Oral Surg, Oral Med and Oral Pathol.* 14:690–703.

Corio RL, Crawford BE, Schaberg SJ. (1976) Benign cementoblastoma. *Oral Surg, Oral Med and Oral Pathol.* 41: 524–30.

Cornelius EA, McClendon JL. (1969) Cherubism – hereditary fibrous dysplasia of the jaws. *Radiology.* 106:136–42.

Correll RW, Wescott WB. (1983) Asymptomatic, ill-defined radiolucent area in the posterior body of the mandible. *J of Am Dent Assoc.* 107:460–1.

Courage GR, North AF, Hansen LS. (1974) Median palatine cysts. *Oral Surg, Oral Med and Oral Pathol.* 37:745–53.

Courtney RM, Kerr DA. (1975) The odontogenic adenomatoid tumor. *Oral Surg, Oral Med and Oral Pathol.* 39:424–35.

Cowan CG. (1980) Traumatic bone cysts of the jaws. *Int J of Oral Surg.* 9:287–91.

Craig RM, Wescott WB, Correl RW. (1984) A well-defined coronal radiolucent area involving an impacted molar. *J of Am Dent Assoc.* 109:612–3.

Cranin AN, Cranin SL, Silbersher HW. (1970) Paget's disease. *Dental Rad and Photogr.* 43:60–4.

Craver LF, Copeland MM. (1935) Changes of the bones in the leukemias. *Arch of Surg.* 30:639–45.

Crawford BE, Weathers DW. (1970) Osteoporotic marrow defects of the jaws. *J of Oral Surg.* 600–5.

Cremin B, Goodman H, Spranger J, Beighton P. (1982) Wormian bones in osteogenesis imperfecta and other disorders. *Skel Rad.* 8:35–8.

Curran J, Collins AP. (1973) Benign (true) cemento-blastoma of the mandible. *Oral Surg, Oral Med and Oral Pathol.* 35:168–72.

Curtis ML, Hatfield CG, Pierce JM. (1973) A destructive giant cell lesion of the mandible. *J of Surg.* 31:705–8.

Dabska M, Buraczewski J. (1968) Aneurysmal bone cyst. *Cancer.* 23:371–89.

Dahlgren SE, Lind PO, Lindbom A, Martensson G. (1969) Fibrous dysplasia of the jawbones. *Acta Otolaryngol.* 68:257–70.

Dahlin DC. (1978) *Bone Tumors, General Aspects and an Analysis of 6,221 Cases.* Thomas, Springfield.

Dahlin DC, Besse Jr. B, Pugh DG, Ghormley RK. (1955) Aneurysmal bone cyst. *Radiology.* 64:56–65.

Dahlin DC, Henderson ED. (1962) Mesenchymal chondrosarcoma. *Cancer.* 15:410–7.

Dalati T, Zhou H. (2008) Gorlin syndrome with ameloblastoma: a case report and review of literature. *Cancer Invest.* 26(10):975–6.

Daley TD, Wysocki GP, Pringle GA. (1994) Relative incidence of odontogenic tumors and oral and jaw cysts in a Canadian population. *Oral Surg, Oral Med and Oral Pathol.* 77:276–80.

Dammer R, Niederdellmann H, Dammer P, Nuebler-Moritz M. (1997) Conservative or radical treatment of keratocysts: a retrospective review. *Br J Oral Maxillofac Surg.* 35(1):46–8.

Darroszewaka A, Ralston SH. (2005) Genetics of Paget's disease of bone. *Clin Sci.* 109:257–63.

Davis RB, Baker RD, Alling CC. (1978) Odontogenic myxoma. *J of Oral Surg.* 36:610–5.

Dayan D, Buchner A, Gorsky M, Harel-Raviv M. (1988) The peripheral odontogenic keratocyst. *Int J Oral Maxillofac Surg.* 17(2):81–3.

de Andrade M, Silva AP, de Moraes Ramos-Perez FM, Silva-Sousa YT, da Cruz Perez DE. (2012) Lateral periodontal cyst: report of case and review of the literature. *Oral Maxillofac Surg.* 16:83–7.

de Lange J, van den Akker HP. (2005) Clinical and radiologic features of central giant cell lesions of the jaw. *Oral Surg Oral Med Oral Pathol Oral Radiol Endod.* 99:464–70.

DeBoom GW, Jenson JL, Siegel W, Bloom C. (1985) Metastatic carcinomas of the mandible. *Oral Surg, Oral Med and Oral Pathol.* 60:512–6.

Deighan WJ, Ashley WW, Lazansky JP. (1956) Complex composite odontoma. *Oral Surg, Oral Med and Oral Pathol.* 9:263–8.

Demicco EG, Deshpande V, Nielsen GP, Kattapuram SV, Rosenberg AE. (2010) Well-differentiated osteosarcoma of the jaw bones: a clinicopathologic study of 15 cases. *Am J Surg Pathol.* 34(11):1647–55.

DeTomasi D, Hann JR. (1985) Traumatic bone cyst: report of case. *J of Am Dent Assoc.* 111:56–7.

Dick HM, Simpson WJ. (1972) Dental changes in osteopetrosis. *Oral Surg, Oral Med and Oral Pathol.* 34:408–16.

Dickson DD, Camp JD, Ghormley RK. (1945) Osteitis deformans: Paget's disease of the bone. *Radiology.* 44:449–70.

DiFiore P, Bowen S. (2010) Cemento-osseous dysplasia in African-American men: a report of two clinical cases. *J Tenn Dent Assoc.* 90:26–9.

Drage NA, Whaites EJ, Hussain K. (2003) Haemangioma of the body of the mandible: a case report. *Br J Oral Maxillofac Surg.* 41:112–4.

Duffy JH, Driscoll EJ. (1958) Oral manifestations of leukemia. *Oral Surg, Oral Med and Oral Pathol.* 11:484–90.

Duinkerke ASH, Van de Poel ACM, Doesburg WH. (1975) Variations in the interpretation of periapical radiolucencies. *Oral Surg, Oral Med and Oral Pathol.* 40:414–21.

Dyson DP. (1970) Osteomyelitis of the jaws in Albers-Schonberg disease. *Br J of Oral Surg.* 7:178–87.

Eisenbud L, Attie J, Garlick J, Platt N. (1987) Aneurysmal bone cyst of the mandible. *Oral Surg, Oral Med and Oral Pathol.* 64:202–6.

el-Hajj G, Anneroth G. (1996) Odontogenic keratocysts. A retrospective clinical and histologic study. *Int J Oral Maxillofac Surg.* 25(2):124–8.

Eliasson S, Isacsson G, Kondell PA. (1989) Lateral periodontal cysts. Clinical, radiographical and histopathological findings. *Int J Oral Maxillofac Surg.* 18(4):191–3.

Epstein JB, Voss NJS, Stevenson-Moore P. (1984) Maxillofacial manifestations of multiple myeloma. *Oral Surg, Oral Med and Oral Pathol.* 57:267–71.

Eugenidis N, Olah AJ, Haas HG. (1972) *Hyperparathyroidism. Radiology.* 105:265–75.

Eversole LR, Leider AS, Nelson K. (1985) Ossifying fibroma: a clinico-pathologic study of sixty-four cases. *Oral Surg, Oral Med and Oral Pathol.* 60:505–11.

Eversole LR, Leider AS, Strub D. (1984) Radiographic characteristics of cystogenic ameloblastoma. *Oral Surg, Oral Med and Oral Pathol.* 57:572–7.

Eversole LR, Rovin S. (1972) Differential radiographic diagnosis of lesions of the jawbones. *Diag Rad.* 105:277–84.

Eversole LR, Sabes WR, Dauchess VG. (1973) Benign cementoblastoma. *Oral Surg, Oral Med and Oral Pathol.* 36:824–30.

Eversole LR, Sabes WR, Rovin S. (1975) Aggressive growth and neoplastic potential of odontogenic cysts: with special reference to central epidermoid and mucoepidermoid carcinomas. *Cancer.* 35(1): 270–82.

Eversole LR, Stone CE, Strub D. (1984) Focal sclerosing osteomyelitis – focal periapical osteopetrosis. *Oral Surg, Oral Med and Oral Pathol.* 58:456–60.

Eversole R, Su L, El Mofty S. (2008) Benign fibro-osseous lesions of the craniofacial complex. A review. *Head Neck Pathol.* 2:177–202.

Fantasia JE. (1979) Lateral periodontal cyst. An analysis of forty-six cases. *Oral Surg, Oral Med and Oral Pathol.* 48(3):237–43.

Farman AG, Nortje CJ, Grotepass FW, Farnam J, Van Zyl JA. (1977) Myxofibroma of the jaws. *Br J of Oral Surg.* 15:3–18.

Farnam J, Griffen JE, Schow CE, Mader JT, Grant JA. (1984) Recurrent diffuse osteomyelitis involving the mandible. *Oral Surg, Oral Med and Oral Pathol.* 57:374–8.

Feinberg SE, Finkelstein MW, Page HL, Dembo JB. (1984) Recurrent "traumatic" bone cysts of the mandible. *Oral Surg, Oral Med and Oral Pathol.* 57:418–22.

Fernández LR, Luberti RF, Domínguez FV. (2003) Radiographic features of osseous hemangioma in the maxillo-facial region. Bibliographic review and case report. *Med Oral.* 8(3):166–77.

Finklestein JB. (1970) Osteosarcoma of the jaw bones. *Radiol Clin of N Am.* 8:425–43.

Finley DB, Franklyn P. (1979) Changes in the skull in acute lymphoblastic leukemia of childhood. *Clin Radiol.* 30:431–3.

Fitzgerald GWN, Frenkiel L, Black MJ, Rochon, L, Baxter JD. (1982) Ameloblastoma of the jaws: a 12-year review of the McGill experience. *J of Otolaryngol.* 11:23–8.

Flax N. (1933) Multiple myeloma. *Am J of Roentgenol.* 29:479–86.

Fordham CC, Williams TF. (1963) Brown tumor and secondary hyperparathyroidism. *N Engl J Med.* 269:129–31.

Formoso Senande MF, Figueiredo R, Berini Aytes L, Gay Escoda C. (2008) Lateral periodontal cysts: a retrospective study of 11 cases. *Med Oral Patol Oral Cir Bucal.* 13(5):E313–7.

Forssell K, Sorvari TE, Oksala E. (1974) An analysis of the recurrence of odontogenic keratocysts. *Proc. of Finn Dent Soc.* 70:135–40.

Frame B, Marel GM. (1981) Paget's disease: a review of current knowledge. *Radiology.* 141:21–4.

Franklin CD, Craig GT, Smith CJ. (1979) Quantitative analysis of histological parameters in giant cell lesions of the jaws and long bones. *Histopathology.* 3:511–22.

Franklin CD, Pinborg JJ. (1976) The calcifying epithelial odontogenic tumor. *Oral Surg, Oral Med and Oral Pathol.* 42:753–65.

Freedman GL, Beigleman MB. (1985) The traumatic bone cyst: a new dimension. *Oral Surg, Oral Med and Oral Pathol.* 59:616–8.

Friedman WH, Schwartz AE. (1974) Brown tumor of the maxilla in secondary hyperparathyroidism. *Arch of Otolarynol.* 100:157–9.

Fries JW. (1957) The roentgen features of fibrous dysplasia of the skull and facial bones. *Am J of Roentgenol.* 77:71–7.

Frommer HH. (2005). *Radiology for the Dental Professional*, 8th edn. Elsevier-Mosby, St. Louis.

Gardner AF, Apter MB, Axelrod JH. (1963) A study of twenty-one instances of ameloblastoma: a tumor of odontogenic origin. *J of Oral Surg.* 21:48–55.

Gardner DG. (1980) The central odontogenic fibroma: An attempt at clarification. *Oral Surg, Oral Med and Oral Pathol.* 50:425–32.

Gardner DG. (1984) The mixed odontogenic tumors. *Oral Surg, Oral Med and Oral Pathol.* 58:166–8.

Gargiulo EA, Ziter WD, Mastrocola R. (1971) Calcifying epithelial odontogenic tumor. *J of Oral Surg.* 29:862–6.

Gee JK, Zambito RF, Argentieri GW, Catania AF, Lumerman H. (1972) Paget's disease of the mandible. *J of Oral Surg.* 30:223–7.

George Jr. DI, Gould AR, Behr MM. (1984) Intraneural epithelial islands associated with a periapical cyst. *Oral Surg, Oral Med and Oral Pathol.* 57:58–61.

Ghosh BC, Huvos AG, Gerold FP, Miller TR. (1973) Myxoma of the jawbones. *Cancer.* 31:237–40.

Giansanti JS, Waldron CA. (1970) Odontogenic adenomatoid tumor. *Oral Surg, Oral Med and Oral Pathol.* 30:69–86.

Gill PW, Leaper DJ, Staniland JR, De Dombal FT. (1973) Observer variation in clinical diagnosis – a computer-aided assessment of its magnitude and importance in 552 patients with abdominal pain. *Meth Inform Med.* 12:108–13.

Gingrass RP, Hinz LE. (1961) Fibrosarcoma of the mandible. *J of Oral Surg.* 19:242–4.

Glasscock ME, Hunt WE. (1974) Giant cell tumor of the sphenoid and temporal bones. *Laryngol.* 84:1181–7.

Goldberg H, Schoffield IDF, Popowich LD, Wakeham D. (1981) Cystic complex composite odontoma. *Oral Surg, Oral Med and Oral Pathol.* 51:16–20.

Goldberg SJ, Friedman JM. (1975) Ameloblastoma: a review of the literature and report of a case. *J of Am Dent Assoc.* 90:432–8.

Golden AL, Foote J, Lally E, Beideman R, Tatoian J. (1981) Dentigerous cyst of the maxillary sinus causing elevation of the orbital floor. *Oral Surg, Oral Med and Oral Pathol.* 52:133–6.

Goldenberg D, Sciubba J, Koch W, Tufano RP. (2004) Malignant odontogenic tumors: a 22-year experience. *Laryngoscope.* 114:1770–4.

Gomez LSA, Taylor R, Cohen MM, Shklar G. (1966) The jaws in osteopetrosis. *J of Oral Surg.* 24:68–74.

Goncalves M, Pispico R, Alves Fde A, Lugao CE, Goncalves A. (2005) Clinical, radiographic, biochemical and histological findings of florid cemento-osseous dysplasia and report of a case. *Braz Dent J.* 16(3):247–50.

Gowgiel JM. (1979) Simple bone cyst of the mandible. *Oral Surg, Oral Med and Oral Pathol.* 47:319–22

Granite EL, Aronoff AK, Gold L. (1982) Central giant-cell granuloma of the mandible. *Oral Surg, Oral Med and Oral Pathol.* 53:240–6.

Greditzer HG, McLeod RA, Unni KK, Beabout JW. (1946) Bone sarcomas in Paget's disease. *Radiology.* 146:327–33.

Greer Jr. RO, Johnson M. (1988) Botryoid odontogenic cyst: clinicopathologic analysis of ten cases with three recurrences. *J Oral Maxillofac Surg.* 46(7):574–9.

Grimes WD. (1979) Radiolucent and radiopaque images of the jaws. *Aust Dent J.* 24:5–12.

Groot RH, van Merkesteyn JP, Bras J. (1996) Diffuse sclerosing osteomyelitis and florid osseous dysplasia. *Oral Surg Oral Med Oral Pathol Oral Radiol Endod.* 81(3):333–42.

Gruskin SE, Dahlin DC. (1968) Aneurysmal bone cysts of the jaws. *J of Oral Surg.* 26:523–8.

Gruss JS. (1974) Hemangioma of the mandible: a case report. *Br J of Oral Surg.* 12:24–32.

Guadagnolo BA, Zagars GK, Raymond AK, Benjamin RS, Sturgis EM. (2009) Osteosarcoma of the jaw/craniofacial region: outcomes after multimodality treatment. *Cancer.* 115(14):3262–70.

Gundlach KKH, Schulz A. (1977) Odontogenic myxoma: Clinical concept and morphological studies. *J of Oral Surg.* 6:343–58.

Gurol M, Burkes Jr. EJ, Jacoway J. (1995) Botryoid odontogenic cyst: analysis of 33 cases. *J Periodontol.* 12:1069–73.

Hadi U, Younes A, Ghosseini S, Tawil A. (2001) Median palatine cyst: an unusual presentation of a rare entity. *Br J Oral Maxillofac Surg.* 39(4):278–81.

Haidar Z. (1975) Fibrosarcoma of the mandible: a case report. *Br J Oral Surg.* 13:78–81.

Hamlin WB, Lund PK. (1967) Giant cell tumors of the mandible and facial bones. *Arch of Otolaryngol.* 86:76–83.

Hamner JE, Scofield HH, Cornyn J. (1968) Benign fibro-osseous jaw lesions of periodontal membrane origin. *Cancer.* 22:861–78.

Handlers JP, Abrams AM, Milder J. (1985) Fibrosarcoma of the mandible presenting as a periodontal problem. *J of Oral Pathol.* 14:351–6.

Harder F. (1978) Myxomas of the jaws. *Int J of Oral Surg.* 7:148–55.

Harris WH, Dudley HR, Barry RJ. (1962) The natural history of fibrous dysplasia. *J of Bone and Joint Surg.* 44A:207–33.

Hastleton PS, Simpson W, Craig RDP. (1978) Myxoma of the mandible. *Oral Surg, Oral Med and Oral Pathol.* 46:396–405.

Hayward AL, Sparkes JJ. (1982) *The Concise English Dictionary.* Omega Books, London.

Hayward JR, Melarkey DW, Megquier J. (1973) Monostotic fibrous dysplasia of the maxilla. *J of Oral Surg.* 31:625–7.

Heikinheimo K, Happonen RP, Forssell K, Kuusilehto A, Virtanen I. (1989) A botryoid odontogenic cyst with multiple recurrences. *Int J Oral Maxillofac Surg.* 18(1):10–3.

Henderson MS. (1924) Chronic sclerosing osteitis. *J of the Am Med Assoc.* 82:945–9.

Hendler BH, Abaza NA, Quinn P. (1979) Odontogenic myxoma. *Oral Surg, Oral Med and Oral Pathol,* 47:203–17.

Henrickson P, Wallenius K. (1974) The mandible and osteoporosis. *J of Oral Rehab.* 1:67–73.

Henriksson CO, Jellman O. (1964) Complex odontoma. *Oral Surg, Oral Med and Oral Pathol.* 18:64–9.

Hertzanu Y, Cohen M, Mendelsohn DB. (1985) Nasopalatine cyst. *Clin Radiol.* 36:153–8.

High AS, Main DM, Khoo SP, Pedlar J, Hume WJ. (1996) The polymorphous odontogenic cyst. *J Oral Pathol Med.* 25(1):25–31.

High CL, Frew Jr. AL, Glass RT. (1978) Osteosarcoma of the mandible. *Oral Surg, Oral Med and Oral Pathol.* 45:678–84.

Higuchi Y, Nakamura N, Tashiro H. (1988) Clinicopathologic study of cemento-osseous dysplasia producing cysts of the mandible. Report of four cases. *Oral Surg, Oral Med and Oral Pathol.* 65(3):339–42.

Hillerup S, Hjorting-Hansen E. (1978) Aneurysmal bone cyst – simple bone cyst: two aspects of the same pathologic entity? *Int J of Oral Surg.* 7:16–22.

Hitchin AD, Mason DK. (1958) Four cases of compound composite odontomes. *Br Dent J.* 104:269–75.

Hivanian AG. (1953) Myxoma of the maxilla. *Oral Surg, Oral Med and Oral Pathol.* 6:927–36.

Hoffer O, Vogel G. (1960) Mixed tumor of the salivary glands of the mandible. *Oral Surg, Oral Med and Oral Pathol.* 13:519–22.

Hoggins GS, Allan D. (1971) Paget's disease of the maxilla. *Br J of Oral Surg.* 9:122–5.

Hong SP, Ellis GL, Hartman KS. (1991) Calcifying odontogenic cyst: a review of ninety-two cases with reevaluation of their nature as cysts or neoplasms, the nature of ghost cells, and sub-classification. *Oral Surg, Oral Med and Oral Pathol.* 72:56–64.

Houston GD, Fowler CB. (1997) Extraosseous calcifying epithelial odontogenic tumor: report of two cases and review of the literature. *Oral Surg Oral Med Oral Pathol Oral Radiol Endod.* 83:577–83.

Huber AR, Nissanka EH, Amaratunge EAPD, Tilakaratne WM. (2007) Clinicopathologic analysis of osteosarcoma of the jaw bones. *Oral Dis.* 13(1):82–7.

Huebner GR, Turlington EG. (1971) So-called traumatic (hemorrhagic) bone cysts of the jaws. *Oral Surg, Oral Med and Oral Pathol.* 31:354–65.

Hunsuck EE. (1968) Osteomyelitis of the mandible. *J of Oral Surg.* 26:529–33.

Iannucci JM, Howerton LJ. (2012) *Dental Radiography Principles and Techniques,* 4th edn. Saunders-Elsevier, Philadelphia.

Ide F, Shimoyama T. (2005) Peripheral odontogenic keratocyst: reportof two cases and review of the literature. *Oral Surg Oral Med Oral Pathol Oral Radiol Endod.* 99(1):71–8.

Ingram FL. (1962) Radiology of tumors of the mandible. *Clinic Rad.* 13:47–53.

Inoue H, Miki H, Oshimo K, *et al.* (1995) Familial hyperparathyroidism associated with jaw fibroma: case report and literature review. *Clinical Endocrinol.* 43:225–9.

Jacobs MH. (1955) The traumatic bone cyst. *Oral Surg, Oral Med and Oral Pathol.* 8:90–4.

Jacobsen HH, Vraa-Jensen G. (1949) Fibrous dysplasia of bone. *Acta Radiol.* 31:1–15.

Jacobson HG. (1985) Dense bone – too much bone. Radiological considerations and differential diagnosis. *Skel Radiol.* 13:97–113.

Jacobsson S. (1984) Diffuse sclerosing osteomyelitis of the mandible. *Int J of Oral Surg.* 11:363–85.

Jacobsson S, Hallen O, Hollender L, Hansson CG, Lindstrom J. (1975) Fibro-osseous lesion of the mandible mimicking chronic osteomyelitis. *Oral Surg, Oral Med and Oral Pathol.* 40:433–43.

Jaffe HL, Lichtenstein L, Portis RB. (1940) Giant cell tumor of bone. *Arch of Pathol.* 30:994–1031.

Jayne EH, Hays RA, O'Brien FW. (1961) Cysts and tumors of the mandible. *Am J of Roentgenol.* 2:292–309.

Jones AV, Craig GT, Franklin CD. (2006) Range and demographics of odontogenic cysts diagnosed in a UK population over a 30-year period. *J Oral Pathol Med.* 35:500–7.

Kaffe I, Ardekian L, Taicher S, Littner MM, Buchner A. (1996) Radiologic features of central giant cell granuloma of the jaws. *Oral Surg Oral Med Oral Pathol Oral Radiol Endod.* 81:720–6.

Kaffe I, Naor H, Buchner A. (1997) Clinical and radiological features of odontogenic myxoma. *Dentomaxillofac Radiol.* 26:299–303.

Kangur TT, Dahlin DC, Turlington G. (1975) Myxomatous tumors of the jaws. *J of Oral Surg.* 11:523–8.

Karabouta I, Tsodoulos S, Trigonidis G. (1991) Extensive aneurysmal bone cyst of the mandible: surgical resection and immediate reconstruction. *Oral Surg, Oral Med and Oral Pathol.* 71:148–50.

Karges MA, Eversole LR, Poindexter BJ. (1971) Antrolith: report of case and review of literature. *J of Oral Surg.* 29:812–4.

Karja J, Rasanen O. (1972) Fibrous dysplasia of the jawbones. *Acta Otolaryngol.* 74:138–40

Karpawich AJ. (1958) Paget's disease with osteogenic sarcoma of maxilla. *Oral Surg, Oral Med and Oral Pathol.* 11:827–34.

Kaslick RS, Brustein HC. (1962) Clinical evaluation of osteopetrosis. *Oral Surg, Oral Med and Oral Pathol.* 15:71–81.

Kaugars GE. (1986) Botryoid odontogenic cyst. *Oral Surg, Oral Med and Oral Pathol.* 62(5):555–9.

Kawai T, Hiranuma H, Kishino M, Jikko A, Sakuda M. (1999) Cemento-osseous dysplasia of the jaws in 54 Japanese patients: a radiographic study. *Oral Surg Oral Med Oral Pathol Oral Radiol Endod.* 87(1):107–14.

Kennett S, Pollick H. (1971) Jaw lesions in familial hyperparathyroidism. *Oral Surg, Oral Med and Oral Pathol.* 31:592–610.

Kerley TR, Schow Jr. CE. (1981) Central giant cell granuloma or cherubism. *Oral Surg, Oral Med and Oral Pathol.* 51:128–30.

Khanna S, Gupta S, Srivastava AB, Samant HC, Khanna NN. (1980) Benign fibro-osseous lesions of the jaw. *Ear, Nose and Throat J.* 59:51–8.

Khosla VM, Korobkin M. (1970) Cherubism. *Am J Dis of Children.* 120:458–61.

Kilgour CS. (1958) Hemangioma of the mandible. *Br J of Plastic Surg.* 10:63–9.

Kirby JW, Robinson ME. (1973) Osteitis deformans of the maxilla. *J of Oral Surg.* 31:64–79.

Kline ST, Spatz SS, Zubrow HJ, Fader M. (1961) Large cementoma of the mandible. *Oral Surg, Oral Med and Oral Pathol.* 14:1421–6.

Kohn WG, Collins AS, Cleveland JL, *et al.* (2003) Guidelines for infection control in dental health-care settings, 2003. *MMWR Recomm Rep* 52(RR-17):1–61.

Komabayashi T, Zhu Q. (2011) Cemento-osseous dysplasia in an elderly Asian male: a case report. *J Oral Sci.* 53:117–20.

Koteshwer K, Pillai KG, Rao S, Nayak RG. (1982) Osteosarcoma of the facial bones. *Int J of Oral Surg.* 12:106–9.

Kragh LV, Dahlin DC, Erich JB. (1958) Osteogenic sarcoma of the jaws and facial bones. *Am J of Oral Surg.* 96:496–505.

Kramer IRH, Pindborg JJ, Shear M. (1992) *WHO Histologic Typing of Odontogenic Tumours*, 2nd edn. Springer-Verlag, Geneva.

Krolls SO, Schaffer RC, O'Rear JW. (1980) Chondrosarsarcoma and osteosarcoma of the jaws in the same patient. *Oral Surg, Oral Med and Oral Pathol.* 50:146–50.

Kruse-Losler B, Diallo R, Gaertner C, Mischke KX, Joos U, Kleinheinz J. (2006) Central giant cell granuloma of the jaws: a clinical, radiologic and histopathologic study of 26 cases. *Oral Surg Oral Med Oral Pathol Oral Radiol Endod.* 101:346–54.

Kusukawa J, Irie K, Morimatsu M, Koyanagi S, Kameyama T. (1992) Dentigerous cyst associated with a deciduous tooth. A case report. *Oral Surg, Oral Med and Oral Pathol.* 73:415–8.

Kuttenberger J, Farmand M, Stoss H. (1992) Recurrence of a solitary bone cyst of the mandibular condyle in a bone graft. *Oral Surg, Oral Med and Oral Pathol.* 74:550–6.

Langland OE, Langlais RP, Preece JW. (2002) *Principles of Dental Imaging*, 2nd edn. Lippincott, Baltimore.

Langland OE, Sippy FH, Langlais RP. (1984) *Textbook of Dental Radiology*. Thomas, Springfield.

LeCornu MG, Chuang SK, Kaban LB, August M. (2011) Osteosarcoma of the jaws: factors which influence the prognosis. *J Oral and Maxillofacial Surg.* 69(9):2368–75.

Legunn KM. (1984) Bilateral occurrence of the lateral periodontal cyst: a case report. *Periodontal Case Rep.* 6(2):56–9.

Lemberg K, Hagstrom J, Rihtniemi J, Soikkonen K. (2007) Benign cementoblastoma in a primary lower molar, a rarity. *Dentomaxillofac Radiol.* 36:364–6.

Li TJ, Yu SF. (2003) Clinicopathologic spectrum of the so-called calcifying odontogenic cysts: a study of 21 intraosseous cases with reconsideration of the terminology and classification. *Am J Surg Pathol.* 27(3):372–84.

Lida S, Fukuda Y, Ueda T, *et al.* (2006) Calcifying odontogenic cyst: radiologic findings in 11 cases. *Oral Surg Oral Med Oral Pathol Oral Radiol Endod.* 101(3):356–62.

Looser KG, Kuehn PG. (1976) Primary tumors of the mandible. *Am J Surg.* 132:608–14.

López-Arcas JM, Cebrián L, González J, Burgueño M. (2007) Aneurysmal bone cyst of the mandible: case presentation and review of the literature. *Med Oral Patol Oral Cir Bucal.* 12:401–3.

Lynch DP, Madden CR. (1985) The botryoid odontogenic cyst. Report of a case and review of the literature. *J Periodontol.* 56(3):163–7.

MacDonald-Jankowski D. (1995) Traumatic bone cysts in the jaws of a Hong Kong Chinese population. *Clin Radiol.* 50:787–91.

MacDonald-Jankowski DS. (2003) Florid cemento-osseous dysplasia: a systematic review. *Dentomaxillofac Radiol.* 32(3):141–9.

MacDonald-Jankowski DS. (2008) Focal cemento-osseous dysplasia: a systematic review. *Dentomaxillofac Radiol.* 37(6):350–60.

Mahomed F, Altini M, Meer S, Coleman H. (2005) Cemento-osseous dysplasia with associated simple bone cysts. *J Oral Maxillofac Surg.* 63(10):1549–54.

Manganaro AM, Millett GV. (1996) Periapical cemental dysplasia. *Gen Dent.* 44:336–9.

Manson-Hing LR. (1980) *Panoramic Dental Radiography*, 2nd edn. Thomas, Springfield.

Manson-Hing LR. (1990) *Fundamentals of Dental Radiography*, 3rd edn. Lea and Febiger, Philadelphia.

Mardinger O, Givol N, Talmi YP, Taicher S. (2001) Osteosarcoma of the jaw – the Chaim Sheba Medical Center experience. *Oral Surg Oral Med Oral Pathol Oral Radiol Endod.* 91:445–51.

Marx RE, Sawatari Y, Fortin M, Broumand V. (2005) Bisphosphonate-induced exposed bone (osteonecrosis/osteopetrosis) of the jaws: risk factors, recognition, prevention, and treatment. *J Oral Maxillofac Surg.* 63:1567–75.

Marx RE, Stern D. (2003) *Oral and Maxillofacial Pathology: a Rationale for Diagnosis and Treatment.* Quintessence, Carol Stream.

Meara JG, Shah S, Li KK, Cunningham MJ. (1998) The odontogenic keratocyst: a 20-year clinicopathologic review. *Laryngoscope.* 108(2):280–3.

Mendenhall WM, Werning JW, Fernandes R, Malyapa RS, Mendenhall NP. (2007) Ameloblastoma. *Am J Clin Oncol.* 30(6):645–8.

Mendes RA, van der Waal I. (2006) An unusual clinico-radiographic presentation of a lateral periodontal cyst – report of two cases. *Med Oral Patol Oral Cir Bucal.* 11(2):E185–7.

Mendez P, Junquera L, Gallego L, Baladrón J. (2007) Botryoid odontogenic cyst: clinical and pathological analysis in relation to recurrence. *Med Oral Patol Oral Cir Bucal.* 12(8):594–8.

Miles DA. (2008) *Color Atlas of Cone Beam Volumetric Imaging for Dental Applications.* Quintessence. Chicago.

Mohammadi-Araghi H, Haery C. (1993) Fibro-osseous lesions of craniofacial bones: the role of imaging. *Radiol Clin North Am.* 31:121–34.

Morgan TA, Burton CC, Qian F. (2005) A retrospective review of treatment of the odontogenic keratocyst. *J Oral Maxillofac Surg.* 63(5):635–9.

Murphey MD, Robbin MR, McRae GA. (1997) The many faces of osteosarcoma. *Radiographics.* 17:1205–31.

Nagpal A, Suhas S, Ahsan A, Pai KM, Rao NN. (2005) Central haemangioma: variance in radiographic appearance. *Dentomaxillofac Radiol.* 34:120–5.

Nakayama E, Sugiura K, Ishibashi H, Oobu K, Kobayashi I, Yoshiura K. (2005) The clinical and diagnostic imaging findings of osteosarcoma of the jaw. *Dentomaxillofac Radiol.* 34:182–8.

Napier Souza L, Monteiro Lima Júnior S, Garcia Santos Pimenta FJ, Rodrigues Antunes Souza AC, Santiago Gomez R. (2004) Atypical hypercementosis versus cementoblastoma. *Dentomaxillofac Radiol.* 33:267–270.

Nase JB, Suzuki JB. (2006) Osteonecrosis of the jaw and oral bisphosphonate treatment. *J Am Dent Assoc.* 137:1115–9.

National Council on Radiation Protection and Measurement. (2003) *Dental X-ray Protection.* NCRP Report 145. National Council on Radiation Protection and Measurements, Bethesda, MD.

National Council on Radiation Protection and Measurement. (2017) *Radiation Protection in Dentistry and Oral and Maxillofacial Imaging.* NCRP Report 177. National Council on Radiation Protection and Measurements, Bethesda, MD.

Odukoya O. (1995) Odontogenic tumours: an analysis of 289 cases. *J Oral Pathol Med.* 24:454–7.

Ogasawara T, Kitagawa Y, Ogawa T, Yamada T, Yamamoto S, Hayashi K. (1999) Simple bone cyst of the mandibular condyle with severe osteoarthritis: report of a case. *J Oral Pathol Med.* 28:377–80.

Ogunlewe MO, Oluseyi FA, Wasin LA, Akinola LL, Olutayo J. (2006) Osteogenic sarcoma of the jaw bones: a single institutional experience over a 21 year period. *Oral Surg Oral Med Oral Pathol Oral Radiol Endod.* 101:76–81.

Oliveira GG, García-Rozado A, Rey RL. (2008) Intraosseous mandibular hemangioma. A case report and review of the literature. *Med Oral Patol Oral Cir Bucal.* 13(8):496–8.

Orsini G, Fioroni M, Rubini C, Piattelli A. (2000) Hemangioma of the mandible presenting as a periapical radiolucency. *J Endod.* 26(10):621–2.

Peltola J, Magnusson B, Happonen RP, Borrman H. (1994) Odontogenic myxoma – a radiographic study of 21 tumours. *Br J Oral Maxillofac Surg.* 32:298–302.

Peñarrocha M, Bonet J, Mínguez JM, Bagán JV, Vera F, Mínguez I. (2006) Cherubism: a clinical, radiographic, and histopathologic comparison of 7 cases. *J Oral Maxillofac Surg.* 64(6):924–30.

Petrikowski GC, Pharoah MJ, Lee L, Grace MGA. (1995) Radiographic differentiation of osteogenic sarcoma, osteomyelitis and fibrous dysplasia of the jaws. *Oral Surg Oral Med Oral Pathol Oral Radiol Endod.* 80:744–50.

Philipsen HP, Reichart PA. (1998) Unicystic ameloblastoma: a review of 193 cases from the literature. *Oral Oncol.* 34(5):317–25.

Philipsen HP, Reichart PA. (2000) Calcifying epithelial odontogenic tumor: biological profile based on 181 cases from the literature. *Oral Oncol.* 36:17–26.

Pynn BR, Sands TD, Bradley G. (2001) Benign cementoblastoma: a case report. *J Can Dent Assoc.* 67:260–4.

Regezi JA. (2002) Odontogenic cysts, odontogenic tumors, fibroosseous, and giant cell lesions of the jaws. *Mod Pathol.* 15(3):331–41.

Regezi JA, Sciudba J. (1993) *Oral Pathology. Clinical-Pathologic Correlations.* Saunders, Philadelphia.

Reichart PA, Philipsen HP. (2004) *Odontogenic Tumours and Allied Lesions.* Quintessence, London.

Rizzoli R, Burlet N, Cahall D, *et al.* (2008) Osteonecrosis of the jaw and bisphosphonate treatment for osteoporosis. *Bone.* 42(5):841–7.

Ruggiero SL, Mehrotra B, Rosenberg TJ, Engroff SL. (2004) Osteonecrosis of the jaws with the use of bisphosphonates: a review of 63 cases. *J Oral Maxillofac Surg.* 62:527–34.

Sadoff RS, Rubin MM. (1990) Fibrosarcoma of the mandible: a case report. *J of Am Dent Assoc.* 121:247–8.

Schafer TE, Singh B, Myers DR. (2001) Cementoblastoma associated with a primary tooth: a rare pediatric lesion. *Pediatr Dent.* 23:351–3.

Schneck DL, Gross PD, Tabor MW. (1993) Odontogenic myxoma: report of two cases with reconstruction consideration. *J Oral Maxillofac Surg.* 51:935–40.

Scholl RJ, Kellett HM, Neumann DP, Lurie AG. (1999) Cysts and cystic lesions of the mandible: clinical and radiologic-histopathologic review. *RadioGraphics.* 19(5):1107–24.

Scuibba JJ, Fantasia JE, Kahn LB. (2001) Tumours and cysts of the jaws. In: *Atlas of Tumour Pathology.* Armed Forces Institute of Pathology, Washington, DC: 26–31.

Shear M, Pindborg JJ. (1975) Microscopic features of the lateral periodontal cyst. *Scand J Dent Res.* 83(2):103–10.

Shigematsu H, Fujita K, Watanabe K. (1994) Atypical simple bone cyst of the mandible. *A case report. Int J Oral Maxillofac Surg.* 23:298–9.

Shimizu M, Osa N, Okamura K, Yoshiura K. (2006) CT analysis of the Stafne's bone defects of the mandible. *Dentomaxillofac Radiol.* 35:95–102.

Sidhu MS, Parkash H, Sidhu SS. (1995) Central giant cell granuloma of the jaws – review of 19 cases. *Br J Oral Maxillofac Surg.* 33:43–6.

Sisman Y, Etoz OA, Mavili E, Sahman H, Ertas Tarım E. (2010) Anterior Stafne bone defect mimicking a residual cyst: a case report. *Dentomaxillofac Radiol.* 39:124–6.

Slootweg PJ. (1992) Cementoblastoma and osteoblastoma: a comparison of histological features. *J Oral Pathol Med.* 21:385–9.

Slootweg PJ. (2009) Lesions of the jaws. *Histopathol.* 54(4):401–18.

Smith MH, Brooks SL, Eldevik OP, Helman JI. (2007) Anterior mandibular lingual salivary gland defect: a report of a case diagnosed with cone-beam computed tomography and magnetic resonance imaging. *Oral Surg Oral Med Oral Pathol Oral Radiol Endod.* 103:71–8.

Smith S, Patel K, Hoskinson AE. (1998) Periapical cemental dysplasia: a case of misdiagnosis. *Br Dent J.* 185(3):122–3.

So F, Daley TD, Jackson L, Wysocki GP. (2001) Immunohistochemical localization of fibroblast growth factors FGF-1 and FGF-2, and receptors FGFR2 and FGFR3 in the epithelium of human odontogenic cysts and tumors. *J Oral Pathol Med.* 30(7):428–33.

Standish SM, Shafer WG. (1958) The lateral periodontal cyst. *J Periodontol.* 29:27–33.

Stavropoulos F, Katz J. (2003) Central giant cell granulomas: a systematic review of the radiographic characteristics with the addition of 20 new cases. *Dentomaxillofac Radiol.* 31:213–21.

Su L, Weathers DR, Waldron CA. (1996) Distinguishing features of focal cemento-osseous dysplasia and cemento-ossifying fibroma. A histopathologic spectrum of 316 cases. *Oral Surg, Oral Med and Oral Pathol.* 82:205–15.

Su L, Weathers DR, Waldron CA. (1997) Distinguishing features of focal cemento-osseous dysplasias and cemento-ossifying fibromas: a pathologic spectrum of 316 cases. *Oral Surg Oral Med Oral Pathol Oral Radiol Endod.* 84(3):301–9.

Su L, Weathers DR, Waldron CA. (1997) Distinguishing features of focal cemento-osseous dysplasia and cemento-ossifying fibromas: a clinical and radiologic spectrum of 316 cases. *Oral Surg Oral Med Oral Pathol Oral Radiol Endod.* 84(5):540–9.

Suljak JP, Bohay RN, Wysocki GP. (1998) Lateral periodontal cyst: a case report and review of the literature. *J Can Dent Assoc.* 64(1):48–51.

Sumer M, Gunduz K, Sumer AP, Gunhan O. (2006) Benign cementoblastoma: a case report. *Med Oral Patol Oral Cir Bucal.* 11:E483–5.

Summerlin DJ, Tomich CE. (1994) Focal cemento-osseous dysplasia: a clinicopathologic study of 221 cases. *Oral Surg, Oral Med and Oral Pathol.* 78:611–20.

Telfer MR, Jones GM, Pell GM, Eveson JW. (1990) Primary bone cyst of the mandibular condyle. *Br J Oral Maxillofac Surg.* 28:340–3.

Thomas DW, Shepherd JP. (1994) Paget's disease of bone: current concepts in pathogenesis and treatment. *J of Oral Pathol and Med.* 23(1):12–6.

Toida M. (1998) So-called calcifying odontogenic cyst: review and discussion on the terminology and classification. *J Oral Pathol Med.* 27:49–52.

Tolar J, Teitelbaum SL, Orchard PJ. (2004) Osteopetrosis. *N Engl J Med.* 351(27):2839–49.

Van Rensburg LJ, Nortje CJ, Wood RE. (1994) Advanced imaging in evaluation of a central mandibular hemangioma. *Dentomaxillofac Radiol.* 23:111–6.

Vieira AP, Meneses Jr. JM, Maia RL. (2007) Cementoblastoma related to a primary tooth: a case report. *J Oral Pathol Med.* 36:117–9.

von Wowern N. (2000) Cherubism: a 36-year long-term follow-up of 2 generations in different families and review of the literature. *Oral Surg Oral Med Oral Pathol Oral Radiol Endod.* 90(6):765–72.

von Wowern N. (2001) General and oral aspects of osteoporosis: a review. *Clin Oral Invest.* 5(2):71–82.

Voytek T, Ro J, Edeiken J, Ayala A. (1995) Fibrous dysplasia and cemento-ossifying fibroma: a histologic spectrum. *Am J Surg Pathol.* 19:775–81.

Waldron CA. (1993) Fibro-osseous lesions of jaws. *J Oral Maxillofac Surg.* 51:828–35.

Wang WC, Cheng YS, Chen CH, Lin YJ, Chen YK, Lin LM. (2005) Paget's disease of bone in a Chinese patient: a case report and review of the literature. *Oral Surg Oral Med Oral Pathol Oral Radiol Endod.* 99:727–33.

Weathers DR, Waldron CA. (1973) Unusual multilocular cysts of the jaws (botryoid odontogenic cysts). *Oral Surg, Oral Med and Oral Pathol.* 36(2): 235–41.

Weber AL. (1993) Imaging of cysts and odontogenic tumors of the jaw. Definition and classification. *Radiol Clin North Am.* 31:101–20.

Whaites E, Drage N. (2013) *Essentials of Dental Radiography and Radiology*, 5th edn. Churchill Livingstone-Elsevier, Edinburgh.

Whitaker SB, Waldron CA. (1993) Central giant cell lesions of the jaws. *Oral Surg, Oral Med and Oral Pathol.* 75:199–208.

White S, Pharoah M. (2009) *Oral Radiology: Principles and Interpretation*, 6th edn. Mosby, St. Louis.

Williams HK, Mangham C, Speight PM. (2000) Juvenile ossifying fibroma. An analysis of eight cases and a comparison with other fibro-osseous lesions. *J Oral Pathol Med.* 29:13–8.

Wong GB. (1992) Large odontogenic myxoma of the mandible treated by sagittal ramus osteotomy and peripheral osteoctomy. *J Oral Maxillofac Surg.* 50:1221–4.

Wuehrman AH, Manson-Hing LR. (1981) *Dental Radiology*, 5th edn. Mosby, St. Louis.

Wysocki GP, Brannon RB, Gardner DG, Sapp P. (1980) Histogenesis of the lateral periodontal cyst and the gingival cyst of the adult. *Oral Surg, Oral Med and Oral Pathol.* 50(4):327–34.

Yousem DM, Kraut MA, Chalian AA. (2000) Major salivary gland imaging. *Radiology.* 216(1):19–29.

Zlotogorski A, Buchner A, Kaffe I, Schwartz-Arad D. (2005) Radiological features of central haemangioma of the jaws. *Dentomaxillofac Radiol.* 34:292–6.

Zolle JE, Neugebauer JE. (2008) *Cone-beam Volumetric Imaging in Dental, Oral and Maxillofacial Medicine.* Quintessence, London.

Index

Page numbers in **bold** refer to Tables and *italics* refer to Figures.

Fundamentals of Oral and Maxillofacial Radiology, First Edition. J. Sean Hubar.
© 2017 John Wiley & Sons, Inc. Published 2017 by John Wiley & Sons, Inc.
Companion website: www.wiley.com/go/hubar/radiology